Pink and Blue

Critical Issues in Health and Medicine

Edited by Rima D. Apple, University of Wisconsin–Madison and
Janet Golden, Rutgers University–Camden

Growing criticism of the U.S. healthcare system is coming from consumers, politicians, the media, activists, and healthcare professionals. Critical Issues in Health and Medicine is a collection of books that explores these contemporary dilemmas from a variety of perspectives, among them political, legal, historical, sociological, and comparative, and with attention to crucial dimensions such as race, gender, ethnicity, sexuality, and culture.

For a list of titles in the series, see the last page of the book.

Pink and Blue

Gender, Culture, and the Health of Children

Edited by Elena Conis, Sandra Eder, and Aimee Medeiros

Rutgers University Press

New Brunswick, Camden, and Newark, New Jersey, and London

Library of Congress Cataloging-in-Publication Data

Names: Conis, Elena, editor. | Eder, Sandra, editor. | Medeiros, Aimee, editor.

Title: Pink and blue : gender, culture, and the health of children / edited by Elena Conis, Sandra Eder and Aimee Medeiros.

Description: New Brunswick, New Jersey : Rutgers University Press, [2021] | Includes bibliographical references and index.

Identifiers: LCCN 2020035576 | ISBN 9781978809888 (cloth) | ISBN 9781978809840 (paperback) | ISBN 9781978809857 (epub) | ISBN 9781978809864 (mobi) | ISBN 9781978809871 (pdf)

Subjects: LCSH: Pediatrics—Social aspects—United States—History. | Sex role in children—United States—History. | Sex differences (Psychology) in children—United States—History. | Gender identity in children—United States—History. | Pediatrics—United States—Psychological aspects—History. | Children—Health and hygiene—United States—History.

Classification: LCC RJ47.7 .P56 2021 | DDC 618.92—dc23

LC record available at https://lccn.loc.gov/2020035576

A British Cataloging-in-Publication record for this book is available from the British Library.

♾ The paper used in this publication meets the requirements of the American National Standard for Information Sciences—Permanence of Paper for Printed Library Materials, ANSI Z39.48-1992.

www.rutgersuniversitypress.org

Manufactured in the United States of America

For our children

Contents

Pink and Blue

Coming of Age Together

Gender and Pediatrics

Aimee Medeiros and Elena Conis

In modern pediatric practice, gender matters.

The first vaccine against human papillomavirus was recommended exclusively to girls for years before it was recommended for boys. Boys receive some behavioral diagnoses—attention-deficit/hyperactivity disorder stands out—far more frequently than girls do. Transgender and gender-nonconforming youth access health care services at lower rates than their cisgender peers do.[1] Perhaps this should come as no surprise, given that pediatric advice about not just disease prevention but also play, sports, sexual activity and behavior, diet, hygiene, and even appearance has consistently taken gender, long constructed in overwhelmingly binary terms, into account over the course of the specialty's history.

This book provides a look at how gender, a sociocultural construct, has served as one of the frameworks for pediatric and children's health care in the United States since the specialty's inception. The book also explores how pediatrics has engaged in molding gender as a pervasive sociocultural concept, from the promotion of cultural gender norms through public health campaigns to the use of therapeutics in the reification of the gender binary construct. Its title—*Pink and Blue*—is intended to reflect the color-coding that has often been used in modern pediatrics and public health when reifying gender norms and gender binarism. Pink stands for girl and blue for boy. Gender appears stable, dichotomous, and naturally linked to sex, and its employment in pediatrics to stand for sex endorses the false perception of the objectivity of gender.

This volume was inspired by a call for "new directions" in the history of pediatrics and child health issued by Alexandra Minna Stern and Howard

Markel nearly twenty years ago in *The Formative Years*, their defining work on the subject, which explored how pediatrics and child's health "have been shaped by, and have shaped, the contours of American society."[2] Their work opened up a discussion about how professionals devoted to the care and treatment of children grappled with such social and cultural constructs as race, gender, sexuality, citizenship, and immigration status from the late nineteenth to the end of the twentieth century. *Pink and Blue* continues this discussion and takes it further, by deploying gender—often in concert with class and race—as the central critical lens for understanding the function of pediatrics as a cultural and social project in modern U.S. history. Gender norms, determined socially and culturally, have long framed how pediatric practitioners interpret their patients' bodies, development, behaviors, and psychological well-being. At the same time, pediatric assessments about gender, at both the individual and population levels, carry a degree of authority in society that makes pediatrics a powerful player in how gender in children is culturally understood.

A core argument of *Pink and Blue* is that there is a dialectical relationship between gender and the medical or health care of children that can be explained, in part, by the fact that modern conceptual understandings of gender and the modern purview of pediatrics came of age together. Specifically, the scientific meaning that gender had slowly accrued beginning in the nineteenth century and that was solidified in the mid-twentieth century closely tracked pediatrics' nineteenth-century emergence and mid-twentieth-century shift to a research-oriented field focused on the monitoring of well children.

By the early twentieth century, the term "gender" (long a grammatical classification) had come into rare colloquial use as a synonym for biological sex.[3] But the term acquired a distinctly scientific valence in the mid-twentieth century, through the work of American psychologists, sociologists, clinicians, and others.[4] Its modern use is often traced to Johns Hopkins University psychologist John Money and colleagues' introduction of the concept "gender role" in 1955, which they defined as signifying "all those things that a person says or does to disclose himself or herself as having the status of a boy or man, girl or woman."[5] (Sandra Eder's essay in this volume elaborates on the nuances of this often cited origin.) The concept's migration from Money's lab in the fifties to increasing clinical use in the sixties and then mainstream use in the seventies was enabled through the binary construct of sex as male or female, onto which preexisting sociocultural notions of specific traits associated with each sex were mapped.[6] This process was punctuated in the seventies and early eighties by the use of "gender" by second-wave feminists, who were eager to separate it from biological sex in order to emphasize the distinction between learned roles and innate biology. Meanwhile, the cultural use of "gender" gave meaning to traits and behaviors observed in the two perceived sexes—male and female—as either appropriate or abnormal. By the eighties and nineties, medicalization of these expected traits and behaviors deemed the "appropriate" ones "healthy" and the "abnormal" ones "pathological." Within half a century, the concept of gender thus came full circle, entering, leaving, and then returning to the sphere of scientific research and therapeutic medicine.

Pediatrics' maturation and development as an area of medical professional specialization helped enable the concept of gender to acquire the scientific layer of meaning that it ultimately came to possess. Modern pediatrics endorsed gendered expectations placed on children by imbuing gender differences and stereotypes—and the treatment of deviations from them—with scientific authority. In part, this was possible because the professionalization of modern pediatrics predated these transformations in the conceptualization and deployment of gender by just a couple of decades.[7] As sociologist Sydney Halpern has argued, pediatric practice underwent a notable shift in the 1930s. Pediatricians adopted responsibility for supervising child development. The well-child visit became the norm. As child and infant mortality rates declined, the temporality of pediatrics shifted more futuristic. By the beginning of the 1940s, when the majority of children in the United States were surviving childhood, pediatrics and children's health campaigns could focus not just on saving lives but also ensuring fulfilled adulthoods. These adulthoods themselves were defined significantly, if not exclusively, by social categorizations, including, gender, race, sexual orientation, disability, and nationality. Such categorical expectations formed a feedback loop that shaped how children's bodies and behavior were perceived and treated.

The pediatric specialty had much deeper roots than this, of course. As Minna Stern and Markel noted, pediatrics began to take shape in the latter nineteenth century, arising from what they call "an imbricated biosocial matrix of concepts, institutions, and disease therapies."[8] These included the late nineteenth-century emergence of the idea that childhood was a biological event unparalleled by others and that children were defined by their distinct patterns of development and disease. These notions themselves stemmed from the broad permeation of Charles Darwin's theories, as well as reports emerging from new orphanages, dispensaries, and children's hospitals. Such institutions created settings in which some doctors began to treat only children and thereby began to conceptualize children's medical needs as distinct from those of adults. The first professional meetings of doctors who cared for children convened in the early

1880s, and before the end of the decade, they had founded their own journal and professional association. The first pediatric textbook, American Pediatric Society founding member Luther Emmett Holt's *The Diseases of Infancy and Childhood*, followed in 1897.[9] Holt's *The Care and Feeding of Children*, a pediatric manual written expressly for mothers, would go on to be published from the 1890s through the 1940s.

The timing of this specialty's professionalization followed an important development in professional Western medicine more broadly, one that would shape the field's ideas about and toward gender generally. From the tail end of the eighteenth century to the height of the Victorian era, the medical field had absorbed and reflected back nineteenth-century perceptions of the distinctions between men and women. These distinctions were forged early in the nineteenth century by, among other forces, anti-Enlightenment sentiment, with its rejection of the notion of equality between the binary sexes; the rise of Christian Evangelicalism and its idealization of patriarchy and dichotomized feminine and masculine traits and behaviors; and capitalist industrialization, which fashioned discipline, professionalism, and productivity as prized masculine traits.[10] Politics, business, science, and medicine became masculine domains defined by the masculine traits of restraint and reason; the home became the feminine preserve, femininity the domain of emotion, modesty, and passivity. Nineteenth-century physicians who emerged predominantly from the white, professional classes absorbed these values and attitudes. In turn, science and medicine adopted the broader social project of maintaining a clear distinction between the male and female sexes. As Victorian-era biomedical knowledge emphasized differences between men and women, it imbued these differences with the objectivity and authority of scientific fact.[11] By the time pediatrics began to emerge as its own distinct area of specialization, American and European physicians had well-documented distinctions between the binary sexes and had thus amply contributed to the social project of maintaining the sharp—and by then scientific—line of demarcation in the male/female binary.

The gender project of Victorian science and medicine deserves more attention in studies of the history and specifically the emergence of the pediatric specialty. At the same time, however, a focus on the specialty's late nineteenth-century emergence may have already come at the expense of deeper historical understanding of how gender—and race, at the very least—operated in the medical care of children before the profession emerged. The emergence of modern pediatrics is often cited as a post–Civil War event, but, in addition to Victorian gender mores, the antebellum medical care and treatment of children—which included the profit-driven treatment of enslaved children, the promotion of citizenship for white children, and the acceptance of race-based disparities in biology and health—was influential in the foundation of the medical specialty. In short, children's health and medical needs were long attended to prior to the formation of the pediatric profession, of course, and the historically gendered and racialized treatment of such children would eventually be imprinted upon the specialty itself.

This is evident, for example, in early nineteenth-century child health treatises that stressed the importance of good health within the framework of citizenship conceived along a boy/girl binary. Mary Palmer Tyler's *The Maternal Physician*, a popular health manual for mothers of infants and young toddlers in the 1810s, offered instructions intended to serve as guideposts for parents tending to children through the epidemics, common ailments, and hazardous conditions that plagued American youth at the time. Tyler's advice to parents played off of predominantly middle-class parental anxieties and societal expectations around rearing future gendered citizens. When championing infant play over restraining limbs, for instance, she suggested that mothers not "immure boys, from a desire to see them look fair and delicate," because what will ultimately be most appealing will be their "courage, strength, and activity."[12] She warned that letting one son's "sport with superior grace the lily hand and diamond ring" will cause them to be effeminate and pusillanimous and that "the poison will quickly pervade" the child's "whole soul."[13] At the same time, she emphasized that girls were to be taught and cared for in a way that would ensure they would grow up to be innocent and demure.

For enslaved children, by contrast, a starkly different set of considerations motivated the care and guidance offered by white experts and physicians. In 1808, when the congressional ban of slave importation went into effect and the future of slavery in the United States became dependent on natural increase, slaveowners increasingly looked to doctors (typically of their own race and class) to help protect their assets. And yet slave infants were born at an average birth weight lower than that of other infants at the time, and young enslaved children were frequently abused or sexually assaulted.[14] They were also malnourished, as they were not considered productive enough to receive the same nutrition as older slaves. Most enslaved children nonetheless worked, often in harsh conditions. Such children's labor, contingent as it was on health, equated to wealth potential for their owners; medical care thus sought to preserve productivity, not shape future citizenship.[15]

The disparities in the histories of children of different races, classes, and citizenship status, itself a theme of this collection, speak to yet another theme in this volume: the relationship between childhood and the economy. The role of the child in American capitalism has evolved over the past two hundred years, with specific implications for the gendered culture of pediatrics. During the late nineteenth and early twentieth centuries, as sociologist Viviana A. Zelizer has shown, the modern, middle-class American child changed from an economically "useless" to emotionally "priceless" family member, bringing forth new sentimental criteria to determine each such child's worth.[16] As the value of the (usually white) middle-class child's labor diminished, their role in consumption began to grow and would continue to grow over the twentieth century.[17] Such children would also come to play a role in their parents' consumption, as the raising of healthy babies and children constituted a set of needs that helped push their parents into the realm of modern consumer culture in the early twentieth century.[18] By the later twentieth century, direct-to-consumer advertising of products for the well child (or, by then, any child) would target parents *and* children; given that children rarely purchase their own goods, marketing needed to motivate the parent as well as the child. In this context, gender-coding became a means of signaling, through colors and gender-specific depictions, the intended user, girl or boy, and the sex-specific benefits that would presumably accrue. By the end of the twentieth century and beginning of the twenty-first century, pediatrics and certain public health campaigns targeting children, as essays in this volume show, would mimic this gendered strategy, hoping to match the success of other dealers in the children's consumer market.

The pediatric specialization's nineteenth-century emergence also coincided with social campaigns that brought attention to infant mortality, broadly, as a social problem best addressed through sanitation and infrastructure. An emphasis on nutrition and malnourishment and bacteriology followed in the last decades of that century, supplanted by national agencies and programs promoting scientific motherhood in the early decades of the twentieth century.[19] By then, the care of children was divvied up between predominantly male pediatricians in the clinic and female social reformers at the societal level. Tension between the two is epitomized by the American Medical Association's opposition to the 1921 Sheppard-Towner Maternity and Infancy Act—a piece of legislation that provided funding for maternity and childcare and whose programs were administered through a staff dominated by female social reformers. The dispute eventually led to the founding of a second professional society for pediatricians, the American Academy of Pediatrics, in 1930. By this time, gender's influence on the structure of children's health care had completed a decisive turn. Tyler's 1818 manual, notably, had opened with an introduction that declared "every mother her child's best physician."[20] A century later, as sociologist Sydney Halpern notes, early practitioners joked at professional meetings about "taking over the traditional functions of neighbors and grandmothers," in the process infusing them with the authority of scientific medicine.[21] This transfer of authority was critical to overcoming what one early practitioner described as "the great trial of my life": the grandmother "probably has had eight children and I have not had any."[22]

Sociocultural concepts are often unstable categories, and gender is no exception. As the editors of this volume, we acknowledge the uniqueness of the present cultural moment, in which the hegemony of gender binarism and conformity is being simultaneously upheld and vigorously contested. Over the arc of the long twentieth century, gender became increasingly homogenized through medical normalization. Transformations in scientific medicine did not counter this shift, and at times they even accelerated it. And yet in the past decade, a series of clinics focusing on gender-affirming care for patients twenty-one years of age and younger have been established across the country. Such clinics aim to provide safe and supportive care for gender-nonconforming and transgender youths, and such care has helped open up questions about the fundamentally gendered culture of pediatrics.

Despite this, the boy/girl binary still serves as an organizing structure in pediatric care and as an influential concept in health research and health campaigns, as Mamo and Pérez, among others, demonstrate in this volume. Halpern noted that pediatrics has always been strongly influenced by ideological currents and social reform movements outside of the medical profession. At the same time, pediatrics is, like any other medical specialization, a status- and market-driven phenomenon achieved gradually by generations of practitioners.[23] The emergence of clinics specializing in the treatment of transgender and nonbinary youth must be understood in the context of this aspect of the specialty's history, too. This volume seeks to bring to light the subtle but still powerful workings of the boy/girl binary in pediatrics, as well as medicine's role in affirming the binary's sociocultural authority and in sanctioning its deconstruction. By interpreting, applying, and reifying gender in various hidden and visible ways throughout the long twentieth century and into the twenty-first century, this volume traces how gender has operated, and still operates, as a clinically and culturally convenient, if problematic, category in the health and medical care of children.

Pink and Blue aims to be the first book to illuminate the complex relationship between cultural notions of gender and pediatric research and practice. Divided into two sections—Clinical Practice and Body Politic—the book considers how gender is produced and applied in the clinic; explores what happens when pediatric knowledge, produced on the basis of gendered assumptions, is applied at a population level; and shows how these two sites are mutually constitutive in producing a particular notion of American childhood, benchmarked against a white, middle-class, heterosexual, capitalist norm. Historians of medicine and public health have analyzed the history of children's health in the United States and examined the critical role of gender in shaping medical norms and practices in this country, but to date, no single volume of scholarship has prioritized the intersection of these lines of inquiry.[24]

The first section of this book, Clinical Practice, examines historical and contemporary examples of how clinical practices and norms control and conceptualize gender in plain sight. In chapter 1, "A Tale of Two Charts," Aimee Medeiros explores the uncontested practice of sex segregating in growth and development data in modern pediatrics. Using the growth chart as a case study, this chapter provides a striking example of how gender was mapped onto a sex binary during the twentieth century, which thereby naturalized its use in scientific medicine. Jessica Martucci's historical analysis of medical and parental attitudes toward young children's sexual self-stimulation, in chapter 2, offers an example of how medical expertise fed, and then pushed back against, cultural assumptions, including gendered ones, that framed children's masturbation as pathological. Some early experts, she found, reserved their harshest treatments for masturbating girls, and even as medical attitudes toward the behavior softened into tolerance, subtle signs of pathologizing judgment persisted.

The child patient's gender was not all that mattered in clinical encounters; practitioner and parental gender influenced such encounters as well. As Hughes Evans shows in chapter 3, the fate of infants with Down syndrome in the mid-twentieth century was decided by tacit agreements between male doctors and pediatricians who explicitly excluded mothers, whom they deemed frail and excessively emotional, from the process. The history sketched by Sandra Eder, in chapter 4, offers a counterpoint from the same era depicting the clinic as a place where new ideas about sex and gender were produced within and through clinical practices and needs. She shows the concerns of and debates among clinicians that led a team of pediatric endocrinologists, psychologists, and psychiatrists to abandon a biological definition of sex in favor of a learned "gender role" in the 1950s, in their clinical encounters with children with divergence of sex development, or intersex.

Jules Gill-Peterson's personal-historical account, in chapter 5, brings aspects of the history in Eder's article up to the present, with its exploration of how trans identity shapes specific forms of encounters with medical gatekeeping from childhood into adulthood. Gill-Peterson offers a history of transgender children's medicalization during the twentieth century. During this time, sex and gender were medically associated with children's plasticity, an inherently racialized notion of how young, white bodies formed and changed through "normal" growth. In chapter 6, "Race and Gender in the NICU," authors Christine Morton, Krista Sigurdson, and Jochen Profit bring this history of racialized, gendered clinical assumptions up to the present, showing how race mapped onto gender to mold practitioner responses to care provided in twenty-first-century neonatal intensive care units. The chapter discusses the emergence in the 2000s of a set of clinical memes, the "wimpy white boy" and "strong Black girl." It discusses their historical roots, their potential role in the "hidden curriculum" of medical training, and implications for the persistence of racialized ideas in medicine and their attendant pernicious effects on access to equal quality of care.

Since the turn of the twentieth century, children's health has been a partly private and partly public endeavor.[25] This volume's second section, Body Politic, explores the operation of gender within the realm of public health, public debate, and policy. In chapter 7, "Masculinity and the Case for a Childhood Vaccine," Elena Conis finds the justification for a mandated, and widely accepted, childhood vaccine in more than a century's worth of medical, government, and popular concern over mumps' various and exclusive effects on men. These included sequelae ranging from mumps-induced "insanity" in individual men to testicular mumps complications among companies of soldiers. In chapter 8, "Weight, Height, and the Gendering of Nutritional Assessment," Andrew Ruis examines how gender operated in early twentieth-century public health nutrition, with a focus on the nutrition classes offered to undernourished children through schools, dispensaries, and other institutions. Ruis argues that gender formed the basis for assumptions about how to motivate children to improve their diets and self-care: boys were encouraged to be healthy so they could be athletic and grow into productive workers; girls were encouraged to eat right so they could be beautiful and grow into their future roles as wives, mothers, and caregivers. In chapter 9, Kathleen Bachynski examines midcentury pediatricians' efforts to promulgate and promote policy to correct for a national trend toward organized children's sports that was largely focused on boys. The American Academy of Pediatrics pushed—largely without success— for intramural, universal athletic programs for young children of both genders in the name of physical fitness and better health for all; Bachynski considers the implications of this history for boys' and girls' sports to the present day.

Longstanding and seemingly ineluctable tensions over children's respective identities as future sexual adults form a current that run through the volume's last two chapters, which follow the younger subjects of earlier chapters into their preadolescent and teenage years. In chapter 10, "Gender and the 'New' Puberty," Heather Munro Prescott notes that gender, race, and sexuality have long framed anxieties related to purportedly premature puberty. Prescott's chapter reveals how adult concerns about the prevailing social order, from the early twentieth century to the present, shaped medical and lay understandings of "normal" adolescent sexual development, as well as the ways in which these norms were strongly gendered. For Laura Mamo and Ashley Pérez, the authors of chapter 11, these gender norms have powerfully reasserted themselves through more than a decade of evolving efforts to promote the human papillomavirus (HPV) vaccine to preteens. Initially, as they show, strongly gendered promotional efforts reflected the underlying assumption of female responsibility for population-level sexual health. Subsequent vaccine promotion campaigns aimed to "de-gender" the vaccine and its target infection in an effort to increase uptake among boys. But gender norms emphasizing female responsibility for sexual health across the life span ultimately reasserted themselves, in the form of more recent HPV vaccination recommendations that applied to female bodies from childhood through adulthood and to male bodies only in childhood.

Although most of the chapters in this volume focus on the past century, they cover more than two hundred years of history. They cover only a small sample of issues and episodes from that history—and yet they make clear the extent to which pediatrics and children's public health played key roles in preparing American children for an adulthood benchmarked against white, middle-class, heterosexual, and capitalist expectations. For all of these children, gender formed another layer of expectation, one that gave specific forms to other features of their anticipated adulthood. This layer was no less foundational, as it dictated the productive roles children were being primed to fulfill, whether through labor, procreation, or both. Gender helped define what health meant for "boys" and "girls": the strength, beauty, and freedom from disease necessary to meet the prevailing heteronormative middle-class expectation to marry a member of the opposite sex, have children, and contribute to the care of those children, the nation, or the economy.

On the most fundamental level, then, pediatric conventions regarding the appropriate traits and behaviors of children were shaped by assumptions about their future roles as gendered adults. The long history of mumps and its vaccine, for example, reveals how mumps threatened boys' and young men's perceived ability to assume their expected roles as the nation's future soldiers, laborers, and fathers. The much shorter history of the HPV vaccine, meanwhile, shows how its use reflected girls' and women's responsibility for sexual health and cancer prevention across both genders. Pediatrics' many metric tools, from the growth chart to the skeletal maturation atlas, developed to assess children's progression along their paths to normal, healthy adulthood, were profoundly shaped by gendered expectations of children and helped perpetuate such gendered expectations into their adulthoods.

At the same time, as the essays herein reveal, pediatric and public health practices reveal anxieties about allowing children to progress too quickly along that path. These concerns are most evident in anxieties about the sexualization of child behavior and attributes, from toddler masturbation to early signs of puberty. Gender marked key distinctions among these anxieties, too. Early twentieth-century warnings about early puberty, as Prescott notes in chapter 10, were stronger for girls than they were for boys. The mother of a masturbating girl in chapter 2 felt it necessary to affirm her daughter's intelligence; the mother of a masturbating boy, by contrast, expressed concern about his corrupting influence on other children. Cultural ideals about female sexual passivity and purity (and a deeply historical association between masturbation and mental health), Martucci points out, help explain the differences in parental response. In chapter 5, Gill-Peterson offers an explanation for childhood as a locus of social norms and anxieties about future sexual identity and behavior. Gender, she argues, emerges through the inherent imagined plasticity of childhood. Importantly, Gill-Peterson notes, plasticity is an imagined feature of white bodies, which explains why white trans and gender-nonconforming children received, historically, clinical attention that children of color did not. The same concept goes some distance in explaining the gendered and racialized contemporary meme applied to infants in intensive care, discussed in chapter 6: the Black, female infant bodies are inherently strong; the white, male, and therefore plastic bodies can be made so through clinical intervention.

Throughout this volume, essays offer examples of those who went against the grain, challenging or refusing gender norms, for either personal or political reasons: the father who wanted, against medical advice, to share with his wife the decision to remove their baby with Down syndrome from the family. The health experts who told parents not to pathologize their toddler's sexual self-stimulation. The pediatric endocrinologists who urged letting patients choose their own sex. The vaccine developers who sought a larger market for a product widely perceived as critical for only the female sex, degendering the target infection, HPV, in the process. But as Mamo and Pérez argue in chapter 11, this only goes so far: responsibility for the sexually transmitted infection's prevention boomeranged back to the female domain despite marketing and public health campaigns that sought to overturn this deeply embedded sociocultural assumption.

This volume's focus is the United States; its subjects are children who are overwhelmingly, but not exclusively, white and usually middle class. This is a legacy of the medical specialty at its late nineteenth-century inception: at that time, pediatric practitioners were predominantly male and white, and they made pediatrics, intentionally or not, in their image and in keeping with their values. Pediatric practices and norms, as Medeiros notes in chapter 1, absorbed and reflected back the deeply bifurcated gendered social order of the day. As a result, myths about children of different genders—and races and classes—were rationalized through American public health and clinical practice focused on the care and treatment of the nation's youngest citizens. As the essays herein illustrate, this legacy persists. To this day, gender's imprint—alongside the imprint of race and class—is legible on everything from sexual attributes and behavior to nutritional advice and vaccination protocols. That the latter examples are linked to the former examples through the operation of gender is the main takeaway from this book.

To be sure, in emphasizing age as a category of analysis, other categories receive less attention than they deserve. Moreover, there is much, including many urgent child health matters, that this volume does not adequately cover. To name just a few: racism, gun safety, autism, obesity, substance dependence, vaccine hesitancy, toxic chemical exposures, behavioral health, border health, neurodiversity, health disparities, climate and health, and the health concerns unique to children living in poverty, in immigrant communities, in undocumented families, and in other contexts that distance them from the benefits—and sometime hazards—of the pediatric clinic and its attendant spaces. Nonetheless, we hope that this book inspires a wide diversity of urgently needed scholarship on how scientific rationalization can perpetuate harmful myths based on the gender, racial, class, and other differences ever evident among American children.

Notes

1. G. Nicole Rider et al., "Health and Care Utilization of Transgender and Gender Nonconforming Youth: A Population-Based Study," *Pediatrics* 141, no. 3 (March 2018): 1.
2. Alexandra Minna Stern and Howard Markel, *Formative Years* (Ann Arbor: University of Michigan Press, 2004), 2.
3. "Gender, n.," in *OED Online* (Oxford University Press), accessed October 4, 2019, http://www.oed.com/view/Entry/77468.
4. David Haig, "The Inexorable Rise of Gender and the Decline of Sex: Social Change in Academic Titles, 1945–2001," *Archives of Sexual Behavior* 33, no. 2 (April 2004): 87–96.
5. John Money, J. G. Hampson, and J. L. Hampson, "Hermaphroditism: Recommendations Concerning Assignment of Sex, Change of Sex and Psychologic Management," *Bulletin of the Johns Hopkins Hospital* 97, no. 4 (October 1955): 284–300.
6. Haig, "The Inexorable Rise of Gender and the Decline of Sex."

7. Quoted phrase in Committee on Pediatric Workforce, "Definition of a Pediatrician," *Pediatrics* 135, no. 4 (April 1, 2015): 780–81.

8. Minna Stern and Markel, *Formative Years*, 3.

9. Minna Stern and Markel, 6–7.

10. Mark S. Micale, *Hysterical Men: The Hidden History of Male Nervous Illness* (Cambridge, MA: Harvard University Press, 2009), 56–57. See also Nancy Leys Stepan, "Race, Gender, Science and Citizenship," *Gender & History* 10, no. 1 (1998): 26–52.

11. Cynthia Eagle Russett, *Sexual Science: The Victorian Construction of Womanhood* (Cambridge, MA: Harvard University Press, 1989).

12. Mary Palmer Tyler, *The Maternal Physician: A Treatise in the Nature and Management of Infants from the Birth until Two Years Old Being the Result of Sixteen Years' Experience in the Nursery Illustrated by Extracts from the Most Approved Medical Authors by an American Matron* (Philadelphia: Lewis Adams, 1818), 277.

13. Tyler, 279.

14. Marie Jenkins Schwartz, *Birthing a Slave: Motherhood and Medicine in the Antebellum South* (Cambridge, MA: Harvard University Press, 2006), 15; Richard H. Steckel, "Women, Work, and Health under Plantation Slavery in the United States," in *More Than Chattel: Black Women and Slavery in the Americas*, ed. David Barry Gaspar and Darlene Clark Hine (Bloomington: Indiana University Press, 1996), 43–62.

15. Steckel, "Women, Work, and Health," 44.

16. Viviana A. Zelizer, *Pricing the Priceless Child* (Princeton, NJ: Princeton University Press, 1994).

17. David Buckingham and Vebjørg Tingstad, eds., *Childhood and Consumer Culture* (Basingstoke, UK: Palgrave Macmillan, 2010).

18. Janet Golden, *Babies Made Us Modern* (New York: Cambridge University Press, 2018), 74.

19. Rima D. Apple, *Perfect Motherhood: Science and Childrearing in America* (New Brunswick, NJ: Rutgers University Press, 2006).

20. Tyler, *The Maternal Physician*, 5.

21. Sydney A. Halpern, *American Pediatrics: The Social Dynamics of Professionalism, 1880–1980* (Berkeley: University of California Press, 1988), 13.

22. Halpern, 166, n. 31.

23. Halpern.

24. There is a sizable literature on the history of children's health and medicine, as well as another on the operation of gender in medicine's history. For further reading on the history of children's health, see, for example, Rima Apple, *Perfect Motherhood: Science and Childrearing in America* (New Brunswick, NJ: Rutgers University Press, 2006); Joan Brumberg, *Fasting Girls: The History of Anorexia Nervosa* (New York: Vintage, 2000); James Colgrove, *State of Immunity: The Politics of Vaccination in Twentieth-Century America* (Berkeley: University of California Press, 2006); Cynthia Comacchio, Janet Golden, and George Weisz, eds., *Healing the World's Children: Interdisciplinary Perspectives on Health in the Twentieth Century* (Montreal: McGill-Queens University Press, 2008); Cynthia A. Connolly, *Children and Drug Safety: Balancing Risk and Protection in Twentieth Century America* (New Brunswick, NJ: Rutgers University Press, 2018); Debbie Doroshow, *Emotionally Disturbed: A History of Caring for America's Troubled Children* (Chicago: University of Chicago Press, 2019); Paula S. Fass and Mary Ann Mason, eds., *Childhood in America* (New York: New York University Press, 2000); Evelynn M. Hammonds, *Childhood's Deadly Scourge: The Campaign to Control Diphtheria in New York City, 1880–1930* (Baltimore: Johns

Hopkins University Press, 1999); Richard Meckel, *Save the Babies: American Public Health Reform and the Prevention of Infant Mortality 1850–1929* (Rochester, NY: University of Rochester Press, 1990); Richard Meckel, Janet Golden, and Heather M. Prescott, eds., *Children and Youth in Sickness and Health* (Westport, CT: Greenwood, 2004); Heather M. Prescott, *A Doctor of Their Own: The History of Adolescent Medicine* (Cambridge, MA: Harvard University Press, 1998). For further reading on gender in the history of medicine and science, see, for example, Ruth Bleier, *Science and Gender: A Critique of Biology and Its Theories on Women* (New York: Teachers College Press, 1997); Anne Fausto-Sterling, *Sexing the Body: Gender Politics and the Construction of Sexuality* (New York: Basic Books, 2000); Julia Grant, "A 'Real Boy' and Not a Sissy: Gender, Childhood, and Masculinity, 1890–1940," *Journal of Social History* 37, no. 4 (2004): 829–51; Bernice L. Hausman, "Do Boys Have to Be Boys? Gender, Narrativity, and the John/Joan Case," *NWSA Journal* 12, no. 3 (Fall 2000): 114–38; Wendy Kline, *Building a Better Race: Gender, Sexuality, and Eugenics from the Turn of the Century to the Baby Boom* (Berkeley: University of California Press, 2005); Beth Linker, *War's Waste: Rehabilitation in World War I America* (Chicago: University of Chicago Press, 2011); Joanne J. Meyerowitz, *How Sex Changed: A History of Transsexuality in the United States* (Cambridge, MA: Harvard University Press, 2002); Jennifer L. Morgan, *Laboring Women: Reproduction and Gender in New World Slavery* (Philadelphia: University of Pennsylvania Press, 2004); Leslie J. Reagan, *Dangerous Pregnancies: Mothers, Disabilities, and Abortion in Modern America* (Berkeley: University of California Press, 2012); Londa Schiebinger, *Nature's Body: Gender in the Making of Modern Science* (Boston: Beacon, 1993); Elizabeth Siegel Watkins, "The Medicalisation of Male Menopause in America," *Social History of Medicine* 20, no. 2 (2007): 369–88.

25. Golden, *Babies Made Us Modern.*

Part 1

Clinical Practice

Chapter 1

A Tale of Two Charts

The History of Gendering Sex-Specific Growth Assessment in Pediatrics

AIMEE MEDEIROS

Growth charts and tables have been important clinical assessment tools in modern pediatrics since its inception. A sex binary—male/female—has always been used to organize and present data featured on this type of diagnostic tool, a framework that predicates a sex differential in growth and development. Rarely questioned, this premise has withstood the evolution of the growth chart. In 2000, the Centers for Disease Control and Prevention (CDC) color-coded its sex-specific growth charts using a gendered color palette from contemporary marketing campaigns targeting children and parents. Charts intended to track the growth of girls were colored pink and the charts for boys were colored blue.[1] This was the first time the CDC color-coded its growth charts based on gender, and it did so without any official explanation or justification.

This essay tells the story of how the gendering of the sex-specific growth charts in 2000 was made possible by the oversaturated, gendered consumer culture of the 1990s as well as the pediatric tradition of using the binary construct of sex when assessing growth. It begins by looking at how using average measurements as health norms in the evaluation of growth in American pediatrics dates back to the end of the nineteenth century, a time when those engaged in anthropometry and medicine were interested in how race, sex, immigration, and nationality factored into a child's development. As population health research continued to pursue all of these lines of interests, sex became the mechanism by which standards were created and presented on tables and charts in clinical medicine, reflecting a larger masculinity project in science at the turn of the twentieth century.[2] Sex segregation kept boys at a particular age safe from being assessed as smaller if averages were derived from data from all children.

Having one set of average measurements used to appraise girls and another to evaluate boys, the sex binary served as a prophylactic for boys and made possible the gendering of the growth charts at the turn of the twenty-first century.

However, to attribute the pink and blue of the CDC charts solely to sex specificity in growth assessment would be misleading, as the coloring of these charts is also a product of the hypergendered children's consumer culture of the late 1990s. At that time, children's worlds were inundated with gendered images, many of which were in hues of pink and blue. In this overmessaged, overgendered consumer culture, the gendered color-coding of the new charts went unnoticed, signifying their ordinariness. This essay concludes by considering the cultural compatibility and medical utility of gendered sex-specific growth charts in an increasingly gender-fluid society.

A Battle of the Sexes

The scientific study of growth and development of children in the United States began in the 1870s with large growth surveys, the first of which was orchestrated by Henry Pickering Bowditch in Boston, Massachusetts. Born in 1840, Bowditch received his medical degree from Harvard and then traveled to France and Germany in 1868, where he studied physiology and worked in laboratories. When he returned to Boston, Bowditch became an assistant professor of physiology at Harvard Medical School and served on Boston's School Committee.[3]

Bowditch was an early proponent for the collection of measurements and assessment of growth in pediatrics. His interest in conducting growth research stemmed in part from a debate in Europe about whether boys and girls grew at the same rate and whether girls were ever bigger than boys during childhood. The dispute began when Belgian statistician and theorist of human variance and averages Adolphe Quetelet suggested that Belgian girls were never taller than boys the same age as them, grew less rapidly than boys, and stopped growing before boys in part because girls had less "vital energy."[4] A prevailing concept at the time, vital energy came from the idea that the body had a limited amount of energy and that if that energy was used in one capacity, say menstruation, then there was less available for another activity, such as education or physical growth.[5] In this regard, Quetelet's observations about girls' subordinate performance to boys were consistent with the wide-held belief at the time that women were weaker than men.[6]

In the same treatise, Quetelet addressed evidence that refuted his idea that girls were always smaller than boys. Growth surveys of children in Manchester and Stockport featured in the first volume of *Factory Reports* reported that working-class girls were superior to their male counterparts in height and weight between the ages of thirteen and fourteen.[7] He argued that these findings were not contrary to his hypothesis; instead, they proved how industrial manufacturing harmed boys and perverted the natural order.[8]

American scientists, including Bowditch, were eager to weigh in on the debate and offer their own findings. In 1872, Bowditch presented a small growth study he had been working on for twenty-five years to the Boston Society of Medical Sciences. His presentation included a chart with two growth curves representing the average measurements of growth in height of twenty-five individuals, twelve males and thirteen females, who were related (most likely to him). The curves were sex specific and drawn in a way so that comparisons could be made, most notably that girls grew faster and were about one inch taller than boys between the ages of twelve and a half and fourteen, when they stopped growing while boys continued to "grow rapidly" until nineteen.[9] According to the *Boston Medical and Surgical Journal*, Bowditch's talk stirred interest in conducting "extended observations" related to differences in growth, perhaps in part because they would have been seen as anomalous to the prevailing theory that school-aged girls were weaker than their male counterparts, especially during menstruation.[10]

In 1875, the Boston School Committee granted Bowditch permission to move forward with a growth survey of pupils in public schools.[11] During the study, close to 24,500 measurements were collected and thousands of interviews with children were conducted.[12] Schools were sent blank forms that would allow them to record a student's name, age, height, weight, and birthplace, along with the nationality of the father and mother and information about parents' occupation. Height and weight measurements were collected by educators or school administrators. The blank forms also included a section for "remarks," where teachers were told to record "any deformity" or if the student was "negro and mulatto." While it is difficult to determine Bowditch's level of interest in how disability or blackness may have influenced growth, or in the children who would have been deemed disabled and/or Black, the omission of these data and possible conclusions in the survey's official report might provide a clue.[13]

At the same time, the quality and quantity of data collected allowed for the Boston growth survey to make meaningful contributions to the field of anthropometry and the debate about growth when it came to the "comparative rate of growth of the two sexes." The survey's findings were similar to those from the Manchester and Stockport studies and Bowditch's smaller study. According to the official report, what was deemed one of the "important results" from the investigation was that boys were taller and heavier than girls until the age of eleven or twelve. Then, for the next two years, girls surpassed boys in weight and height. However, the report argued that girls' supremacy over boys in stature was brief, as "boys then acquire and retain a size superior to that of girls who have now nearly completed their full growth."[14] Although it is challenging to tell how Bowditch felt about his findings confirming that girls were bigger than boys for a period of time during childhood, the report's emphasis on its fleeting nature and boys' ultimate superiority over girls is noteworthy. While couching boys' inferiority to girls in male dominance might have lessened the observation's blow to masculinity, the research did show that girls were bigger than boys for a period of time during development. This finding would have been problematic for those involved in scientific medicine at the end of the nineteenth century, as most research of the time supported the theory that men were superior to women. From evolution studies to exercise science, scientific research was engaged in a project of proving that there were differences between men and women and that women were naturally weaker than men.[15]

Innocuously presenting the sex differential in stature at ages eleven to thirteen gained importance in the 1880s, when pediatricians began adopting data from growth surveys and repurposing them as healthy average measurements to be used to assess children in clinical practice. At the second annual meeting of the American Medical Association's section on children's diseases in 1881, Bowditch argued that "it seems probable that the accurate determination of the normal rate of growth in children will not only throw light upon the nature of diseases to which childhood is subject but will also guide us in the application of therapeutic measures."[16] Pediatrician and textbook author Luther Emmett Holt followed Bowditch's advice and featured two tables with average measurements from growth surveys serving as health norms in his hugely influential textbook, *The Diseases of Infancy and Childhood.*[17] The sex binary was used to present these norms in two tables, a table on the "Weight of Older Children" and a "Table showing Weight, Height and Circumference of the Head and Chest from Birth to the Sixteenth Year." In the table featuring average measurements of weight for children, columns were organized by the sex binary girl/boy. The other table, which depicted the healthy norms of weight, height, chest, and head measurements from birth to sixteen, used the sex binary to divide data line by line, with averages for boys in bold typeface.[18] Although there seemed to be some degree of edits made to the chapter addressing growth and development with each of the textbook's most influential editions, the use of the girl/boy sex binary to present healthy norms in growth and development was always used and never justified.[19] Hence, the nondisputed sex specificity of these healthy norms shielded boys in early adolescence from being assessed by measurements from girls who were on average bigger than them. It also perpetuated the idea that boys were on average bigger than girls throughout childhood.

Setting Sex-Specific National Standards

In the first half of the twentieth century, there were a handful of growth charts and tables for clinicians to choose from, with the two most popular being the Baldwin-Wood and Woodbury tables.[20] Part of the reason there was no preferred set of charts or tables was due to a failure to agree upon the "norms or the manner in which evaluations should be made." However, the majority of these growth assessment tools did share one characteristic. Most of them were sex specific.[21]

In 1949, sex specificity in growth assessment received a national endorsement when the Joint Committee on the Health Problems in Education of the National Educational Association and American Medical Association released the instructional booklet, *Physical Growth Record*. Meant to standardize the recording and interpreting of height and weight measurements of school children, *Physical Growth Record* featured growth charts generated by Dr. Howard V. Meredith of the Iowa Welfare Research Station and Dr. Harold C. Stuart of the Department of Maternal and Child Health at the Harvard School of Public Health. The booklet, and the charts in it, came in two versions: one for girls and one for boys.[22]

An article by Dr. Howard V. Meredith accompanied the publication of the *Physical Growth Record*. In it, Meredith described how the booklets were made, their intended use, and their shortcomings. According to Meredith, the process was seamless, as all parties involved agreed early on that "separate booklets would be prepared for boys and girls"; "the charts on pages 2 and 3 of the booklets would begin at age 4 years and extend to age 18"; they would be easy to read; the Joint Committee would sponsor and distribute them; and Meredith would write an article in conjunction with their release.[23] He then elaborated on the best use of the booklets and their potential in assessing the height and weight of children.

While Meredith did not elaborate on the collective choice to make the booklets sex specific, he did address a deficit with the data used to create the charts—a lack of diversity—which he felt could result in an inaccurate evaluation of a child's stature. He explained how the height and weight measurements for the Stuart-Meredith charts had come from several hundred "white children of northwest European ancestry" living in Iowa "under better-than-average conditions from the standpoints of nutrition, housing, and healthcare."[24] Next,

Meredith asked, "Are the normative materials presented in the charts appropriate for use in any North American school? More specifically, are they validly
employed in schools whose pupils are drawn from the unskilled-laborer class,
or from districts largely populated by families of Italian, Mexican, or Japanese
ancestry?" In responding to his own questions, Meredith suggested that most
"school physicians and pediatricians consider it preferable to evaluate children
of low socio-economic status" and from "ethnic groups" with measurements
collected from their respective populations.[25]

Meredith did not elaborate on how the sex specificity of the data could also
distort the growth assessment of a child. In fact, there was no mention as to why
the charts and booklets were sex specific. Indeed, these charts allowed for identical measurements to be evaluated differently due to the sex of a child. For
example, according to the charts, a twelve-year-old girl who was 58 inches
tall would be assessed as "moderately short," while a boy of the same age and
height would be seen as "average."[26] It appears that the sex specificity of the
charts shielded early adolescent boys from the sex differential confirmed by
Bowditch and others in the late nineteenth century. In the case of these growth
charts, the sex binary played a significant role in evaluating the stature of a
child as it continued to protect boys from the bigger sizes of girls their same age.

Maintaining the perception that boys were always bigger than girls would
have been particularly important at this time. In postwar America, the threat of
communism was depicted as sinister and real. The strength of the United States
was measured in part by the health of its citizens and the maintenance of daily
life. Small-stature boys would have signaled a weakness in modern American
society that would have made the nation susceptible to a takeover by the Sovi-
ets or their allies.[27]

The Stuart-Meredith charts served as the de facto national set of growth
charts in the United States from 1949 until the mid-1970s, when the National
Center for Health Statistics (NCHS) decided to construct "new growth charts for
today's children."[28] One of the first steps in this process was the creation of an
advisory group tasked with making decisions about data selection and the formatting of the charts. Based on the published report, the group seemed to have
quickly identified what data to use, as the national Health Examination Surveys
had recently collected thousands of measurements. But because the surveys did
not include children aged zero to two, the group decided that NCHS should pull
data from a well-respected longitudinal study conducted by the Fels Research
Institute of 867 middle-class, formula-fed, white Americans living near Dayton,
Ohio. While not necessarily representative of the majority of American children,

these data would serve as norms that would promote healthy living and living standards, or so the experts argued.[29]

The advisory group also discussed the format of the charts. During deliberations, it contemplated the possible need for a series of charts that were race based. In the end, the group was of the opinion that "one set of data for all races would be sufficient for practical purposes, despite the small but actual differences in body measurements noted among racial groupings." The same type of consideration was not given to the sex specificity of the charts. According to the published report, the advisory group never discussed or questioned the rationale behind formatting the growth charts using the male/female sex binary.[30]

In 1976, the NCHS released a series of fourteen sex-specific growth charts consisting of smoothed growth curves of plotted percentile points based on distributions of body size (weight, height, and head circumference) attained at specific chronological ages from birth to eighteen years of age. These charts were to be used for nutritional screening, public health assessments of populations of children, and clinical standards for children and infants in the United States. They laid the foundation for the CDC/NCHS charts, which were released one year later (1977), as well as the 1978 NCHS/World Health Organization (WHO) charts.

In use for almost twenty-five years, these CDC/NCHS/WHO charts set national and international growth standards and further normalized the boy/girl sex binary in children's health, as the sex of the child remained centralized in growth assessment. Even when these charts came under scrutiny, their sex specificity remained unquestioned. Some critics found the variety in sample size and measurement type (cross-sectional and longitudinal) problematic. For example, as preferences in the feeding of infants shifted from formula to breastmilk in the United States, the infant charts, which were based on measurements from formula-fed infants, no longer seemed suitable for assessing infants' growth and development accurately.[31] Many argued the charts needed updating in order to remain effective in evaluation.

In the 1990s, the federal government decided it was time to begin the process of replacing the NCHS growth charts with new ones. Beginning in December 1992, the Division of Health Examination Statistics at NCHS hosted the first of four workshops to discuss concerns and "solicit recommendations on approaches that could be taken in the revision process."[32] At the first workshop, experts from "various Federal agencies and academic institutions" came up with a series of questions about the project, including how the older charts should be updated, whether there should be ethnic-specific charts, what data should be used to develop charts for infants, and whether the charts should be made available online. Workshops two, three, and four took on specific topics from this list: a specific infant study, the use of data from low birthweight infants, and the trend of an increase in bodyweight among children, adolescents, and adults, respectively. But no workshop or expert seemed to question the charts' sex specificity.[33]

After about a decade of discourse and development, the new set of CDC growth charts was released, in 2000. The CDC's official report accompanying these charts concluded that they were "developed with improved data and statistical procedures" and that "health care providers now have an instrument for growth screening that better represents the racial-ethnic diversity and combination of breast- and formula-feeding in the United States." It also instructed that the 2000 CDC growth charts were to replace the old set "when assessing the size and growth patterns of infants, children, and adolescents."[34]

Similar to the NCHS charts, the new set was sex specific, which meant that sex continued to play an important role in growth assessment. For example, based on the 2000 CDC individual "length-for-age" charts for boys and girls, an eighteen-month-old boy who was 30 inches would be placed on the lowest curve, which represents the third percentile, while a girl the same age would be seen as closer to average, since she would be one curve away from the one representing average growth in girls. Even though the children were identical in height, the girl would be considered nearer a normal growth pattern than the boy due to her sex assignment at birth.[35] This also meant that boys would be seen as viable candidates for stature-promoting therapeutics at taller heights than girls.

These new sex-specific charts were, for the first time, color-coded based on the perceived gender of their intended subjects, with the charts for girls colored pink and those for boys colored blue. The official report accompanying the new charts neglected to address the decision to color-code the charts, an omission that might point to how noncontroversial this change seemed at the time.[36] While the long-standing practice of sex specificity in growth assessment made the charts' gender makeover possible, the hypergendered children's consumer culture of the late 1990s and early 2000s made it probable. In fact, the pink and blue hues of the growth charts failed to catch media attention, unlike other new elements, most notably the addition of a set of body mass index charts, or BMI charts, meant to monitor the increased bodyweight of children in general and curb the national obesity epidemic, one child at a time.[37]

The ubiquity of gender in modern children's consumer culture made the gendered color schema of the CDC sex-specific growth charts probable. Leading up to the charts' release, gender had played an increasing role in marketing campaigns targeting children and their parents since the deregulation of children's television programming in the 1980s, a federal move that opened the door for advertisers to market products direct-to-child. By the end of the decade, most children's shows looked more like *He-Man and the Masters of the Universe* than *Sesame Street*. In this environment, gendering tactics, such as color-coding, were seen as effective marketing tools for conveying who was best suited for the product and for selling more merchandise.

He-Man and the Power of Television

Before the era of deregulation, federal agencies tried to protect young television viewers from unbridled capitalism with varying levels of success. For example, in 1974, the Federal Communications Committee (FCC) took a stand when it recommended "advertising limits of 12 minutes per hour on weekdays and 9.5 minutes on weekends" and strongly urged the implementation of what it called the "separation principle": a ban on "any form of program-related product promotion."[38] The television industry disagreed with the FCC and failed to act, which led the Federal Trade Commission (FTC) to endorse a ban on all television advertising directed at children younger than eight. Believing that the FTC had crossed a line with this restriction, Congress voted to "rescind the FTC's jurisdiction to regulate unfair advertising," leaving the television industry to self-regulate.[39] Within a short time, this played a part in the emergence of a strongly gendered color-coding in children's consumer culture.

Mattel was the first toy manufacturer to take advantage of opportunities made possible by the deregulation of children's television programs. In 1983, it introduced the toy-based animated television program series, *He-Man and the Masters of the Universe*. The company had a design team develop a toy line with a powerful and extramuscular main character who could take on anything, who was literally "the most powerful man in the universe." The show, which aired after school, targeted boys with muscular characters, swords, and magic. The program stirred immediate opposition, but nonetheless, "within a year He-Man toys were the second-best sellers in the industry."[40] Other toy manufacturers took notice and came up with their own made-for-TV marketing schemes that exploited exacerbated gender stereotypes for profit.[41]

By 1984, the commodification of children's television programming was bolstered by the FCC's decision to abandon all quantitative commercial guidelines and to reinterpret product-related programming as an innovative funding technique rather than a predatory practice. In three years, the number of toy-based cartoons increased by 30 percent.[42] Each TV series was accompanied with its own line of toys and merchandise. It was typical for shows to target either boys (*He-Man, G.I. Joe*) or girls (*She-Ra, My Little Pony 'n Friends*) through the use of gendered characters, storylines, and color palettes.[43] Gender coding was also not exclusive to children's television programming; rather, it infiltrated multiple cross-pollenating mediums, including print, film, textiles, and toys during this time period.[44] For example, the influential toy section of the Sears catalog underwent a gendered makeover. In 1975, 2 percent of toys featured in the catalog were explicitly marketed to either girls or boys. Decades later, "gendered toys made up half of the Sears catalog's offerings."[45]

Just as He-Man had taken over children's television in the 1980s, a series of successful Disney princesses—*The Little Mermaid, Beauty and the Beast, Aladdin, Pocahontas*, and *Mulan*—ushered in what has been labeled "girlie-girl culture" in the 1990s.[46] This feminine turn of children's consumer culture came with its own official color: pink.[47] Pink reigned supreme as marketing campaigns utilized what was perceived to be a "strong association" between gender and certain color palettes. Bold colors conveyed maleness while pastel colors signaled femininity. When single colors were used, companies chose pink, lavender, and purple to target girls and sometimes blue to target boys, albeit inconsistently. As online shopping grew in popularity, gendered color-coding migrated to the new medium.[48] A study of the gender marketing of toys on the Disney Store website found that "85% of toys that had red, black, brown, or gray as their most predominant color were for 'boys only,'" while "86.2% of toys that were pink were for 'girls only.'"[49] Pink proved to be a powerful and direct signal to consumers about which products were specifically being marketed to girls and their parents.

It was during the height of the use of gender messaging in marketing campaigns targeting children and their parents that the CDC released its new set of color-coded, sex-specific growth charts, making them cultural artifacts of a time when the binary construct of gender served as a valuable marketing tool. Indeed, at the onset of the twenty-first century, gender was used to organize the shelves of toy stores, sell clothing, and inspire the reclassification of male pop music groups to boy bands.

As of 2020, these charts were still in use, even as the gender wave in consumer culture had waned.[50] In 2015, Disney stopped categorizing children's costumes by gender. That same year, Target abandoned gender-specific aisles in its toy section. In 2016, the White House Council on Women and Girls hosted a conference "aimed at shifting the way media and toys present gendered images to young people."[51] And in 2018, Mattel stopped using gender to classify toys. The company launched the first gender-neutral doll a year later.[52] According to a *Time* magazine article, Mattel's new Creatable World doll "can be a boy, a girl, neither or both." Gender fluidity was gaining traction as it offered an alternative to the rigid gender binary that was in vogue during the 1990s and 2000s.

The Future of Sex-Specific Growth Charts

What is the future of gendered, sex-specific growth charts, especially in an increasingly gender-nonconforming society? A case study from a 2008 clinical casebook can help answer this question. In *Affirmative Mental Health Care for Transgender and Gender Diverse Youth*, readers learn of a prepubescent gender-nonconforming child with a difference/disorder of sex development (DSD) condition, in a case report titled "'I'm Here to Get Taller and Because I Want to Be a Boy': A Case of Down-Turner Mosaicism in a Prepubescent Gender-Nonconforming Child."[53] This case study was selected by the authors because while most individuals experiencing gender dysphoria (GD) do not have a co-occurrence of DSD, there is a higher prevalence of GD in individuals with DSD. The authors wanted to ensure that even with a co-occurrence of DSD, the child's gender identity would be supported by mental health care professionals.[54]

The case concerns a child who had been assigned female at birth and was starting to assert a male identity. During an unrelated visit, the child was evaluated by an endocrinologist due to her short stature. Test results revealed she had a 45,X/47,XY,+21 Down-Turner mosaic karyotype, meaning that in the "20 cells tested, 12 cells had 45,X chromosomes and 8 had 47, XY,+21 chromosomes." While individuals on average have forty-six chromosomes in all cells of their body, this child did not. One cell line was missing a X or Y chromosome (45,X) while the other cells had an extra chromosome (47,XY). Based on these findings, the seven-year-old child was technically both male and female at the cellular level.[55]

After the child received an official diagnosis of Turner syndrome (TS) with Y chromosome mosaicism, the family was then referred to a multidisciplinary Turner Clinic, where they had multiple sessions with a psychologist. The child started transitioning to a boy shortly after. This included a new name, Sam, and new pronouns, he/him/his. Sam also received growth hormone (GH) therapy, which he perceived as part of his transition because of the popular belief that boys are taller than girls. However, his Turner syndrome diagnosis actually made him a viable candidate for this height-promoting therapy because the Food and Drug Administration had approved GH therapy for children experiencing short stature due to Turner syndrome beginning in the 1990s.[56] For Sam, however, GH therapy was gender affirming because it promised height.

Although not mentioned in the case study, a decision would have needed to have been made as to which sex-specific growth chart would be used to assess

Sam's growth, even though no chart exists that is based on data from a specific subset representative of Sam: a transgender boy with TS with Y chromosome mosaicism. Selecting the girl's chart could be psychologically damaging, since its pink hues would not be considered gender affirming. The boy chart would be equally problematic. While its blue color might align with Sam's gender identity, he was never clinically assigned a male. While clinicians might not anticipate Sam's growth data to follow along featured growth curves on any existing chart given his diagnoses and gender identity, they likely would have desired to track his development as they adhered to gender-affirming clinical practices.[57]

While this case might appear unique, it does highlight the potential trappings of the use of gendered sex-specific growth charts in a nonbinary world. According to pediatrician Stanley Vance, growth assessment is complicated "when it comes to [the use of] charts in gender diverse populations" because "there is insufficient data and no guidelines with how to use" them. Vance, an adolescent medical specialist in eating disorders, said, "The most important thing I can do as a provider is for my interactions with the patient to be gender-affirming, but I also need to detect anything medically concerning. There is a lack of long-term studies looking at growth in transgender youth populations who are starting blockers and hormones."[58]

As of 2020, growth charts made specifically for transgender youth, including those receiving hormone therapy, did not exist. Instead, what medicine had to offer was gendered sex-specific growth charts that espoused the sex binary and linked specific genders to sexes through color-coding. While in clinical settings, health professionals often select which charts will be used to track the growth of the patient, choosing one that does not align with a child's gender identity could cause psychological harm. Could this not be true for all children? It is time to reconsider the use of sex specificity in growth assessment and to rid gender messaging from growth charts.

Notes

1. Robert J. Kuczmarski, National Center for Health Statistics (U.S.), and National Health and Nutrition Examination Survey (U.S.), *CDC Growth Charts for the United States: Methods and Development* (Hyattsville, MD: Dept. of Health and Human Services, Centers for Disease Control and Prevention, National Center for Health Statistics, 2002), 19–44.
2. Mark S. Micale, *Hysterical Men: The Hidden History of Male Nervous Illness* (Cambridge, MA: Harvard University Press, 2009), 56–57.
3. Aimee Medeiros, *Heightened Expectations: The Rise of the Human Growth Hormone Industry in America* (Tuscaloosa: University of Alabama, 2016), 26.
4. M. Adolphe Quetelet, *A Treatise on Man and the Development of His Faculties* (Edinburgh: William and Robert Chambers, 1842), 58.

5. Patricia Vertinsky, "Exercise, Physical Capability, and the Eternally Wounded Woman in Late Nineteenth Century North America," *Journal of Sport History* 14, no. 1 (1987): 12.

6. Vertinsky, 7.

7. H. P. Bowditch, *The Growth of Children* (Boston: A. J. Wright, 1877), 4.

8. Qutelet, *A Treatise on Man*, 114–15.

9. "Report of Medical Societies," *Boston Medical and Surgical Journal* 87 (1872): 435.

10. "Bibliographic Notices," *Boston Medical and Surgical Journal* 90 (1874): 626.

11. Bowditch, *The Growth of Children*, 4.

12. Bowditch, 7.

13. Bowditch.

14. Bowditch, 35.

15. Michael S. Kimmel, "Men's Response to Feminism at the Turn of the Century," *Gender and Society* 1, no. 3 (1987): 261–83; William F. Pinar, "The 'Crisis' of White Masculinity," *Counterpoints* 163 (2001): 321–416. See also Vertinsky, "Exercise."

16. H. P. Bowditch, "The Relation between Growth and Disease," in *The Transactions of the American Medical Association* (Philadelphia: Collins, 1881), 373.

17. L. Emmett Holt, *The Diseases of Infancy and Childhood* (New York: D. Appleton and Company, 1898), 15–22.

18. Holt, 19–20.

19. "Growth and Development of the Body," in L. Emmett Holt, *The Diseases of Infancy and Childhood* (New York: D. Appleton and Company, 1897, 1902, 1905, 1907, 1909, 1911, 1916, 1919, 1922, 1926, 1933), pages vary.

20. Robert L. Jackson and Helen G. Kelly, "Growth Charts for Use in Pediatric Practice," *Journal of Pediatrics* 27, no. 3 (1945): 215–29.

21. Jackson and Kelly, 216.

22. Howard V. Meredith, "Physical Growth Record for Use in Elementary and High Schools," *American Journal of Public Health* 39 (1949): 878–85.

23. Meredith, 873.

24. Meredith.

25. Meredith, 884.

26. Meredith, 880–81.

27. Marilyn Irvin Holt, *Cold War Kids: Politics and Childhood in Postwar America, 1945–1960* (Lawrence: University of Kansas Press, 2014), 27–28.

28. Peter V. Hamill, *NCHS Growth Curves for Children* (Hyattsville, MD: U.S. Department of Health, Education, and Welfare, 1977), 1.

29. Hamill, 1

30. Hamill, 1.

31. Kuczmarski et al., *CDC Growth Charts for the United States*, 1–3.

32. Kuczmarski, 187.

33. Kuczmarski, 188–90.

34. Kuczmarski, 1.

35. Kuczmarski, 21–22.

36. Kuczmarski, 19–44.

37. "Child Growth Charts Updated," *New York Times*, May 31, 2000, A18. Sally Squires, "Keeping Tabs on Budding Flab: New Charts for Children Can Help Identify Weight Problems," *Washington Post*, May 31, 2000, A1.

38. Bonnie A. Lazar, "Under the Influence: An Analysis of Children's Television Regulation," *Social Work* 39, no. 1 (1994): 70.

39. Lazar, 69.

40. Lazar, 70.
41. Lazar.
42. Lazar, 71.
43. Rachel Aschcroft, "The 12 Best 80s Cartoons," https://www.eightieskids.com/the-12 -best-80s-cartoons/.
44. Aschcroft.
45. Elizabeth Sweet, "Toys Are More Divided by Gender Now Than They Were 50 Years Ago," *Atlantic*, December 9, 2014, https://www.theatlantic.com/business/archive /2014/12/toys-are-more-divided-by-gender-now-than-they-were-50-years-ago /383556/.
46. Peggy Orenstein, *Cinderella Ate My Daughter: Dispatches from the Front Lines of the New Girlie-Girl Culture* (New York: Harper Paperbacks, 2012).
47. Orenstein.
48. Carol Auster and Claire S. Mansbach, "The Gender Marketing of Toys: An Analysis of Color and Type of Toy on the Disney Store Website," *Sex Roles: A Journal of Research* 67 (2012): 377.
49. Auster and Mansbach, 381.
50. Maya Rhodan, "The White House Takes Aim at Toys That Perpetuate Gender Ste-reotypes," *Time*, April 6, 2016, https://time.com/4283487/white-house-toys-gender -stereotypes/.
51. Rhodan.
52. Eliana Dockterman, "'A Doll for Everyone': Meet Mattel's Gender-Neutral Doll," *Time*, September 25, 2019, https://time.com/5684822/mattel-gender-neutral-doll/.
53. Diane Chen, Courtney A. Finalyson, Elizabeth Leeth, Elizabeth B. Yerkes, and Emi-lie K Johnson, "'I'm Here to Get Taller and Because I Want to Be a Boy: A Case of Down-Turner Mosaicism in a Prepubescent Gender-Nonconforming Child," in *Affir-mative Mental Health Care for Transgender and Gender Diverse Youth*, ed. Aron Jans-sen and Scott Leibowitz (Cham, Switzerland: Springer, 2018), 91–106.
54. Chen, et al., 92.
55. Chen, et al.
56. Aimee Medeiros, *Heightened Expectations: The Rise of the Human Growth Hormone Industry in America* (Tuscaloosa: University of Alabama, 2016), 2.
57. Fabio Bertapelli et al., "Growth Curves for Girls with Turner Syndrome," *Biomed Research International* 2014 (2014): 108.
58. Dr. Stanley Vance, "Re: The Use of Growth Charts in Pediatric Transgender Care," message to Aimee Medeiros, June 6, 2019, email.

Chapter 2

"A Habit That Worries Me Very Much"

Raising Good Boys and Girls in the Postwar Era

Jessica Martucci

In 1956, Mrs. G, like many other mothers in the postwar years, reached out to ask for help from Dr. Benjamin Spock, the era's foremost pediatrician and parenting advice guru. She shared a problem that had been weighing heavily on her mind. "I have a Boy [of] 19 months, and he has a habit that worries me very much."[1] She went on, "He will lay on the floor on his blanket or teddy bear, or anything, and make up and down motions. At first I just thought it was something new . . . but later it became very apparent that there is more to it than that. I didn't know there were sex feelings that early, and I just don't know what to do about it. . . . Anything can bring it on, looking at a book on his stomach, or laying on the couch, or playing with his sister on the floor." She was particularly concerned about the dynamic between her son and older daughter, who "laughs when he is doing it." "I am really quite unhappy about it," she confessed, "and almost dread company, I am so wound up watching him. . . . Maybe you could write something about it, I would be for ever thankfull [sic]."[2]

One year later, in 1957, another mother—Mrs. P, exasperated for similar reasons about the behavior of her seventeen-month-old daughter—also wrote to Spock for advice. "About 6 months ago," she wrote, just shy of her first birthday, her daughter, whom Mrs. P described as "healthy, normal," and "quite smart for her age," began engaging in some activities that Mrs. P found troubling. She noticed that her daughter liked to squat "down on her hands and knees" and would then rock "back and forth." It wasn't so much the behavior in and of itself that distressed Mrs. P; instead, it was her belief that her daughter was "getting some sort of a satisfactory feeling from this motion and gets quite angry when you try to distract her attention." The mother was somewhat relieved to note that "she does not touch or play with herself" directly, but she was distressed enough about this pleasure-seeking behavior to consult with her pediatrician, whose advice was to "ignore it." Mrs. P, however, could not let it go. By the time she wrote to Spock, she was convinced that the behavior was "getting worse instead of better." "I have read all of your articles in the [*Ladies Home*] *Journal* and have also read your *Child Care* book and find no answer for the problem I seem to have . . . I would be deeply indebted if you could possibly help me."[3]

Buried in the hundreds of mothers' letters in the archives of Benjamin Spock at Syracuse University, these stories about infants masturbating stand out. Masturbation has a long history of being shrouded in taboo, secrecy, shame, and guilt.[4] But these parents' concerns over sexual behaviors in their infants suggest that there may have been something unique playing out in the postwar years when it came to the intersection of child development, pediatrics, gender, sexuality, and parenting. What lay behind these mothers' concerns? What role, if any, had pediatricians played in shaping their concerns? And how might broader cultural ideas and concerns about childhood, gender, and sexuality in this period have shaped these mothers' perspectives and their children's experiences?

This essay places these letters into a broader context in order to better understand these worries and examines what role pediatric experts, like Spock and his predecessors, may have played in the creation and mitigation of these perceived family crises. While medical experts helped pathologize masturbation during the modern era, by the early twentieth century, medical concern on the subject began to wane. The retreat of medical interest in childhood masturbation stemmed in part from shifts in scientific understandings of human development and sexuality that were well under way by the early twentieth century. As child psychology experts increasingly accepted masturbation as a normal part of life, however, cultural anxieties around the practice persisted. While no longer believed to be the cause of "mental degeneracy" or blindness by experts, masturbation in young children continued to sound moral alarms, particularly for mothers who were, as the century wore on, increasingly tasked with raising emotionally healthy and socially well-adjusted children.[5] In the midst of these shifts, mothers encountered a changing postwar landscape in which expectations of sexual pleasure and obligation sat at the heart of ideas about marriage and family life. Raising a well-adjusted child in this era increasingly meant guiding that child through their development into a stable heterosexual adulthood that conformed appropriately to gendered ideas about the passive, contained female and the active, experienced male.

Inventing the Solitary Vice

Numerous scholars over the years have tackled the rise of social, moral, and medical concerns with masturbation that occurred in Western societies between the mid-eighteenth and mid-twentieth centuries.[6] Although any sexual activity that occurred outside of procreative purposes has long been frowned upon in Judeo-Christian religious traditions, most historians point to the pathologization of masturbation as a starting point for the modern era's distaste for the practice.[7] In this well-established narrative, the anonymously published text, *Onania: or, the Heinous Sin of Self-Pollution* (1710), helped mark the beginning of two centuries of medico-moral panic over the idea of seeking sexual pleasure solo.[8] Concerns about the health effects of masturbation mingled with the rising influence of the medical profession at the time. As the behavior came under the jurisdiction of physicians, they issued warnings about side effects such as stunted growth, moral and mental degeneration, loss of reproductive virility in adulthood, and all manner of debility and mental infirmity.[9]

Scholars have also shown that despite important changes and developments in medical science and practice over two centuries, medico-moral anxiety over masturbation seems to have remained fairly consistent, even if the justification for such concern has changed somewhat over time. Persisting fears of depleting one's nervous and procreative energies enveloped young and old, men and women well into the twentieth century.[10] Yet while most scholars who have written on the subject acknowledge that physicians and moral reformers alike were concerned about the practice in men, women, adolescents, and very young children, most of the scholarship has focused on the ideas, concerns, and meanings of masturbation panic on boys and young men.[11] Very little attention has been devoted to the subject of masturbation in girls and women, and where it has, the subject often appears only as a minor subplot.[12] Also, while doctors and advice authors frequently mentioned infants when they wrote about masturbation, there has been no dedicated analysis of how parents or physicians thought about or approached the matter in the very young child and infant.[13] While there is much to be written on the subject of women and girls of all ages, this essay focuses on how ideas about childhood, sexuality, and gender shaped midcentury perceptions of and attitudes toward self-stimulation in the very young—infants and toddlers under the age of three.

By the end of World War I, the medical profession began to relinquish some earlier claims that masturbation caused, or represented, a pathology.[14] It was also during this period that psychology and psychiatry began to assert greater dominion over knowledge about sexuality in mainstream society.[15] Together, alongside work by scientists like Alfred Kinsey, a new gestalt emerged in the postwar years in which sexuality beyond the bounds of procreative sex became increasingly naturalized—even if it remained somewhat suspect.[16] The culprits of pathology by the postwar years increasingly became the guilt, fear, and anxiety that society inflicted upon everyone for "natural," pleasure-seeking sexual activities, rather than the actual act of masturbation. However, if medico-moral fears about the sexual practices of adults, and even adolescents, shifted during this period, what about those for young children? An analysis of mother's letters and childrearing advice from throughout this time suggests that the moral focus and center of agency in infant masturbation moved from the child to the mother.[17] At the same time, pediatricians withdrew their interest in treating masturbation behaviors as a pathology. This left mothers to navigate the era's new gendered expectations about psychosexual development in their very young children, alone.

Medical Ideas about Masturbation in Infancy

The advice literature on masturbation from the mid-nineteenth through the mid-twentieth century provides important context for understanding the meaning these behaviors held for families. This history reveals that parents and physicians had long been tasked with the burden of identifying and addressing masturbation in children. However, letters, advice literature, and medical writings from the postwar era also show that as concerns over the physical health effects of masturbation subsided by the twentieth century, interventions for addressing the issue in the very young child shifted in focus over time from the infant to the mother.

Written in the 1860s by Alfred Vogel, professor of clinical medicine at the University of Dorpat in Russia, the internationally successful *Diseases of Children* informed generations of physicians who joined the developing field of pediatrics at the turn of the twentieth century. On the subject of masturbation, Vogel left no doubt that it was a serious health problem that could strike children at any age. Vogel was most concerned about it in boys, who, he warned, could quickly become emaciated and anemic, and if left unaddressed, the practice could cause them to remain "backward in their bodily . . . and mental development" and their eyelids to turn "brownish or bluish in color; they have apathetic expression[s] . . . and [they developed] flaccid muscles."[18] The younger the age of onset, the more serious the situation, as Vogel believed this would make masturbation a far more difficult habit to break as time wore on. Vogel reported that it had been seen in children as young as eleven months. Yet despite pointing out its existence in infants, Vogel focused almost exclusively on concerns about older children and suggested causes including exposure to other children in boarding schools and other institutional settings, "heavy feather beds," meat, alcohol, and "obscene pictures and stories." The treatments he recommended included constant parental vigilance, hard mattresses, secrecy on the matter, social isolation, and of course swift and severe punishment.[19]

Following the tradition of Vogel, L. Emmett Holt, pediatrician and head of Babies Hospital in New York, in 1897 published *Diseases of Infancy and Childhood*, which went through a series of subsequent editions that stretched through 1940. His medical manual similarly advised physicians to give serious attention to any child caught engaging in masturbation, which he believed could destroy their health. Unlike Vogel, however, Holt focused far more attention on masturbation in the very young. Although he acknowledged it was "more frequent after the eighth or ninth year" and was "especially seen" in the ages between twelve and fifteen, he stressed in the opening paragraph of his passage on masturbation that it was "not uncommon even in infancy."[20] He added that "many cases have been observed during the first year, and some as early as the seventh and eighth month."[21] He had seen many cases for himself as an attending physician in Babies Hospital: "within the last three years at least half a dozen cases have been under observation in children under two years old, some of them most intractable ones."[22]

In a later edition of his textbook, Holt suggested that there were two types of infants who engaged in these behaviors. First were those who did so due to some sort of "local cause," such as a physiological irritation, or due to the teachings of what he referred to as a "vicious nurse." In these cases, a cure could be expected with the right amount of attention. The second type, however, was far less treatable in Holt's opinion. For this group, he observed, it might be a sign of mental "degeneration," and "it is usually hopeless."[23] Holt urged early and swift action: "it is usually a simpler matter to stop it in infants and in young children," he wrote, "as they can be more easily controlled and more closely watched than those who are older."[24] To do this, Holt embraced punishments, as well as technological and medical interventions. "Corporal punishment is often very useful in very young children . . . under three years old," he wrote.[25] The least invasive interventions ranged from mechanical hand restraints, to tying the infant's legs to the sides of the crib, to other immobilizing devices like leg splints and, of course, constant surveillance.

For the more persistent cases, Holt spared no modern medical aid, advocating everything from hypnosis to surgical procedures that included circumcision in boys to clitoral circumcision in girls and even "cauterization of clitoris" in girls who proved to be "obstinate cases."[26] Unlike the more typical etiology of masturbation in adolescents, which Holt claimed was far more common in boys than in girls, in infancy, he remarked that "it is, in my experience, much more common in girls than in boys."[27] As a result, many of his more severe treatments for very young children were geared toward girls. Holt recommended the use of blistering treatments on the thighs and vulva and strongly advised against horseback riding.[28] If all else failed, he recommended the child be sent away from home and kept away from other children, suggesting a stint in the country under the care of a "trustworthy" nurse.[29] Holt's approaches, some of the harshest and most medically involved, were published through the first nine editions of his book, until 1925. Undoubtedly, they continued to have consequences for the ways in which pediatricians approached the issue and the broader cultural attitudes that influenced parents' ideas on the matter.[30] A modestly toned-down 1933 edition of Holt's volume maintained much of the same advice from earlier versions, omitting only the most severe "blistering" treatments.[31]

Nurtured by the shifting philosophies of Progressive-era reformers and child-savers, the idea that children were essentially innocent and deserving of protection, but in need of guidance, wound its way into the burgeoning fields of infant psychology and child development.[32] In this literature, the emphasis on self-stimulation focused on processes behind the formation and prevention of habits. As historian Kathleen Jones has written, "Because the child's character was pliable, regulation of the environment, especially the child's family life, was deemed essential."[33] As the cult of nurture grew, advice to mothers on the subject grew, too. Dedicated to "The Young Mothers," Dr. Elisha Mather Sill's 1913 publication, *The Child: Its Care, Diet and Common Ills*, noted that masturbation was a very widespread practice, one that "may not be recognized by the mother until it has continued for some time."[34] Sill was a well-known physician specializing in childhood diseases who practiced through Cornell's Medical College in Ithaca, New York, before settling in New York City's Good Samaritan Hospital by 1919.[35] Inattentive or permissive mothers might miss dangerous signs of masturbation, he warned, and children who developed this habit could become "pale, sleep poorly, [and grow] . . . easily tired, have dark rings under the eyes, often complain of headaches, are very quiet, have little animation, and do not care to associate with other children."[36] If allowed to continue, he cautioned, they "may even develop melancholia and mental weakness, insanity, or epilepsy."[37] He therefore urged mothers to be vigilant for symptoms of the "condition," including flushed face, "rigidity of the body and lower extremities, followed by relaxation, more or less exhaustion, and often perspiration."[38] In cases in which "the hands are used they should be tied about each wrist with a bandage which passes back of the neck and is tied in front, and which should be long enough to allow free use of the arms and yet short enough to prevent the hands from reaching the genitals."[39] Finally, he suggested the use of mittens such as the "Hand-I-Hold" celluloid baby mitts—marketed originally to thwart thumb sucking and skin scratching. The mitts, he suggested, could be useful in preventing genital touching as well.[40]

The 1914 and 1921 editions of the U.S. Children's Bureau's *Infant Care* guide, also aimed at mothers, adopted a similar approach, suggesting that while masturbation was a "common habit among children," mothers should definitely make "every effort . . . to break it up as soon as possible, as it grows worse if left uncontrolled."[41] Written by Mary Mills West, a college-educated mother who had raised five children, the *Infant Care* guide drew heavily on Holt's work, popularizing it for a wider audience.[42] Despite this, West made the work her own, softening some of Holt's more abrasive approaches. On the issue of infant masturbation, for example, she encouraged mothers to seek medical guidance in case there was some underlying irritation or medical condition. Her 1914 guide advised that careful hygiene, including attentive diapering and bathing, could generally resolve the issue. If it didn't, however, West urged mothers to take decisive action to prevent the behavior from becoming a "habit." Bad habits, like thumb sucking, "crying without cause," and masturbation, all required physical intervention lest they turn into lifelong problems.[43] West advised using "a thick towel or pad . . . to keep the thighs apart while the baby is asleep, and the hands may be restrained by pinning the nightgown sleeves loosely to the lower sheet when putting the baby down for the night."[44] Never, she cautioned, leave "such a baby" alone; "constant and patient watchfulness on the mother's part, are required to break up this habit."[45] Although still concerned with the seriousness of the problem, the 1921 edition of the *Infant Care* guide attempted to further soften approaches and stepped back from some of Holt's most severe recommendations. West wrote that "punishment is worse than useless" for babies and that it would only confuse them and exacerbate the problem.[46] Mothers were to walk an increasingly fine line between taking the condition seriously while still addressing it in a way that did not negatively interfere in their child's development.

By the end of the 1920s, even the idea of restraining an infant's movement to reduce self-stimulation became medically passé. In her 1929 book, *Building the Baby: The Foundation for Robust and Efficient Men and Women*, nurse and educator Carolyn Van Blarcom declared that "the day is long since past when it was believed that the practice caused feeblemindedness, insanity, or mental or physical breakdowns," and anyone who chose to "scold, threaten, shame, or scare the baby" would only "do him much more harm than he is doing himself."[47] Still, despite stating that it was a "common practice among children," she offered advice on how to refocus a child's attention toward other activities—exercise, play with other children, long and hot baths, and a toy to take to bed might keep the baby busy and distract him from focusing his attention "upon himself."[48] If all else failed, however, she remarked that "the young baby who masturbates should have his hands put outside the bedclothes at night."[49] Self-stimulation may have no longer been considered disastrous for an infant's health, but it remained a cause for concern lest a child fail to grow out of it.

By the 1940s, few physicians or health experts expressed serious medical concern over infant masturbation, although the old medico-moral anxieties persisted.[50] Holt's work, republished in 1940, continued to fuel lingering apprehensions. Even when experts themselves could offer no clear medical reason for alarm, however, many continued to categorize self-stimulation in infants as undesirable due to the potential for long-term effects on psychosexual adjustment. New York University pediatrics professors Ruth and Harry Bakwin, for example, approached the topic with little medical concern. Their progressive tone on the subject, however, sat in tension with other, more familiar aspects of their advice. Their 1942 *Psychologic Care during Infancy and Childhood*, aimed at educating mothers and future mothers, matter-of-factly stated that "parents should be assured that manipulation of the genitals during infancy is not harmful and may be disregarded."[51] They also explicitly condemned "the practice of scolding" and "frightening" a child with "tales of dire consequences" and argued that it "is much more harmful than the habit itself," causing shame and resentment in the child.[52] Along with other notable midcentury figures such as Spock, Spock's mentor C. Anderson Aldrich, and the Yale Child Study Clinic's Arnold Gesell, the Bakwins were prominent in the movement to integrate the latest in infant psychology and behavioral research into the pediatric toolkit.[53] But they included their section on masturbation under the heading "Sexual Disturbances" and noted that harm in the "moral and emotional spheres" could arise if practiced habitually.[54] Despite repeatedly stressing masturbation's "normality," the Bakwins provided several pages on how mothers ought to manage, control, and ultimately stop it from happening. And although they dismissed mechanical restraints as useless and harmful, they advocated the use of pharmaceutical sedatives such as "sodium bromide" or "phenobarbital" at night so that the child would fall asleep quickly and not have time for anything else.[55]

The Bakwins' discussion of how to stop the behavior departed subtly but notably from the advice of earlier eras. In encouraging parents to avoid shaming or guilting the child, they suggested that the behavior itself was not actually pathological—instead, the pathology was produced in the child's moral and psychological development as a result of their mother's inappropriate reactions. Their treatment recommendations, therefore, consisted of two approaches: (1) avoiding the situation altogether by removing opportunities for self-stimulation to occur and (2) focusing on the parents themselves, who, they advised, needed to acquire a "moral and intellectual understanding" of their child as an autonomous, psychosexual being. In the Bakwins' writing, a firmer shift toward holding the parents, particularly the mother, accountable for managing these situations in a scientifically informed and rational way is evident. Increasingly, mothers were expected to nurture *appropriate* psychosexual development in their children in order to avoid adulthoods characterized by sexual and social dysfunction. The Bakwins also emphasized that masturbation was most likely to become a habit only in those children who "lead an uninteresting, lonely life," so mothers were asked to not only instill their child with a feeling of "self-confidence" but also provide an active and stimulating mental life to stave off sexual abnormalities.[56]

When Spock published his bestselling *Commonsense Book of Baby and Child Care* in 1946, he shifted away from acknowledging these infant behaviors as sexual at all. Spock included "masturbation" in the book's index, but underneath the entry, he listed "see Handling the Genitals," a much less morally and emotionally fraught way to describe it. "In the infant [any exploration of this kind is] . . . wholesome curiosity," the entry began.[57] Rather than pathologizing or even sexualizing the behavior or the child, Spock explained how routine it was for infants to "discover their genitals," likening it to when they first "discovered their fingers and toes."[58] The potty-training child "explores himself with definite curiosity, for a few seconds at a time," he wrote.[59] Don't worry, he reassured his readers, "this won't come to anything or start a bad habit. You can distract him with a toy if you want, but don't feel that you've *got* to."[60] In fact, he continued, "it's better not to give him the idea that he is bad, or that his genital is bad. You want him to go on having a wholesome, natural feeling about his entire body."[61] Interfering in this "natural" developmental process of self-discovery, he argues, "may have bad results later."[62]

Spock later referred to these harmful effects by speaking to parents on a generational level: "Most of us heard in childhood the threat that masturbation would lead to insanity. This belief is untrue. What's wrong with telling a child that masturbation will make him sick, or injure his genitals, or mark him as an evil person?"[63] Aside from being false, he continued, these stories could damage a sensitive child's sexual development. Such a child may "develop such a morbid fear of anything sexual that he grows up maladjusted, afraid, or unable to marry or have children."[64] Here, Spock spelled out quite clearly what the

Bakwins had only managed to imply—self-stimulation behaviors were a typical part of a healthy infant's normal development, marking a critical moment in their journey to properly embracing their gender and (hetero)sexual identity later on. Spock and his likeminded peers, influenced by the theories of Freud but also increasingly inspired by the era's containment ideology, helped emphasize that it was the mother's responsibility to carefully watch over the infant with only the gentlest and most nonjudgmental guidance. As Mrs. P's pediatrician put it, the best thing a mother could do was to "ignore it."[65]

Despite Spock's popularity and success, not all of his contemporaries agreed with his naturalistic approach to infant sexual development. A survey of the literature published in 1956 by Drs. Milton Levine and Anita Bell identified a 1953 work by Ruth and Harry Bakwin, which continued to stress the subject of prevention, including hand restraints, tying the legs apart in the crib, and amphetamines.[66] A 1951 childrearing advice manual authored by pediatricians Harry R. Litchfield and Leon H. Dembo similarly stated that masturbation in young children was a natural and harmless occurrence, made harmful only by "the guilt feelings associated with the act."[67] Yet they, too, offered advice to mothers on how to manage it, recommending that "if the infant is seen masturbating, the thing to do is to interrupt the act by separating the thighs or removing the hands from that area of the body."[68] At the forefront of progressive changes in developmental pediatrics, Spock was in many ways in a league of his own when it came to his advice, but by the 1950s, even those who continued to express concern over the behavior embraced the idea that only the most gentle guidance from the mother was the best method for changing it.[69]

The Letters in Context

Euro-American ideas about masturbation underwent an important shift between the late nineteenth century, when the germ theory of disease began to gain real acceptance, and the 1930s, when Freud's psychoanalytic theories gained prominence in Western thought. The fundamental nature of this change, as historian Thomas Laqueur explains, was from a medical understanding of masturbation in which it was believed to be a serious matter of health, to a perspective in which it instead was understood by experts as a natural part of human psychosexual development. "By the 1930s," claims Laqueur, "masturbation had . . . become medically benign. . . . Gone were the outlandish claims about disease [from earlier eras]. . . . Gone were efforts to terrorize children and adults into stopping."[70] Under the umbrella of Laqueur's broader narrative, however, smaller stories unfold. By the postwar years, for example, medical emphasis on early infancy as a critical period of development coupled with widespread cultural anxieties about gender roles and homosexuality to incite concern about infantile masturbation among child development experts and mothers alike even as the behavior itself was increasingly understood and accepted as "natural."

By the 1940s, the idea that self-stimulation was a universal and natural part of development in infancy had begun to infiltrate popular parenting discourse. At the same time, mothers in the 1950s had become increasingly aware of the developmental milestones that pediatric experts used to identify and track "normal" growth.[71] When it came to day-to-day living, mothers often found that matching up their own children's behaviors and abilities with what they were *supposed* to be doing (according to the experts) turned out to be far more subjective than many hoped it would be.[72] Driven into states of high anxiety by the high stakes and rigidity they found in advice manuals, mothers sent letters to experts by the thousands in search of clarity and insight into the singular peculiarities of their own children.[73]

Despite medical advice to the contrary, parental skepticism around genital manipulation abounded, fueled by decades, if not centuries, of moralistic medical tales of debility, insanity, and a life of failure for those unable to resist temptation. Scholars have suggested that at least some of what motivated these persisting anxieties were the pressures felt (particularly keenly in the middle class) to raise children who would maintain or surpass the social standing of their parents. As sociologist Nicola Kay Beisel has written, the history of moral crusades reveals that reformers have long sought "to protect children from vice," often in response to middle-class parents' fears that moral failures could "render children unfit for desirable jobs and social positions."[74] Historians, too, have examined connections between socioeconomic class and parental anxieties about morally suspect behavior in children.[75] While many postwar Americans experienced greater prosperity than their parents had, they nonetheless confronted a rapidly changing labor market and economy.[76] Historian Peter Stearns has noted, for example, that the rise of the service economy in the United States during these years put increasing pressure on parents to raise children who possessed the social skills necessary for success.[77] In this historical moment, then, parents increasingly fretted over their children's popularity and invested more and more time and effort into nurturing their kids' emotional and social health.[78]

Pediatricians' willingness to accept and define appropriate sexual development as part of normal human development more broadly did little to ease the burden of anxiety on parents in this period.[79] Mothers, in particular, experienced heightened pressures to guide their children's emotional, psychological, and even sexual development through scientifically educated parenting approaches. Tasked with this responsibility, mothers were routinely cast as fail-ures for either stifling their children's normal development by being "overbear-ing" or by neglecting it and allowing their children to fall prey to moral dangers.[80] If a mother mishandled a child's early sexual development, experts warned that the repercussions could be dire—the child could grow up to be an unwed mother, an emasculated ill-adjusted man, or a lesbian.[81] The specter of homo-sexuality was an issue of paramount concern during the 1940s and 1950s.[82] Pal-pable fears of raising gay sons or lesbian daughters rumbled just beneath the surface of much of the discourse around infant sexual development. This pres-sure to avoid creating sexual difference or deviance in their own infants is clearly visible in mothers' letters to Spock.[83]

Many parents, however, also found the idea that their infants could be sex-ual beings, even developing ones, to be profoundly disturbing. The innocence of childhood had long depended, particularly for girls, on the cultural belief that sexuality was *not* a part of childhood.[84] It was easy enough for a physician to write about infant sexual development in a removed textbook or childrearing manual; it was quite another thing for a parent who spent hours of intimate time with their baby to accept that there was anything *sexual* about it. As one mother wrote in frustration to Spock, "The world has had about all the Freudian half-truths it can stomach," adding "it certainly takes no great powers of observa-tion to note that the baby is not motivated by sex."[85] The combination of these pressures and ideas exacerbated parental anxieties about masturbation. While educated and enlightened parents during this period would have recognized that these behaviors had their place in "normal" infant development, they also knew that, as the Bakwins had stressed, *how* one handled these issues would have lasting impacts.

Laqueur has also observed that over the course of the twentieth century, concerns over female masturbation markedly increased while masturbation in boys became further naturalized. This is certainly reflected in the childrearing advice literature and is even recognizable in these mothers' letters. Although one writes about her son and the other about her daughter, the letter written about the son is devoted largely to how his actions might influence and corrupt her other children, particularly her daughter. In the letter from the mother about her daughter's behavior, she carefully notes that her child is extremely intelli-gent and, if anything, above average in her development. One can only guess at why she felt it was important to add these details, but given the historical asso-ciation between masturbation and mental disorders, it seems reasonable to sug-gest that she highlighted her daughter's mental acuity in order to allay potential concerns that her behavior might indicate an underlying abnormality. Female sexual desire that transgressed cultural ideals of passivity and purity increasingly served as a marker of mental pathology in the medicalizing landscape of nineteenth- and twentieth-century America.[86] Although the postwar years were rife with anxieties about male sexuality, too, concerns about female sexuality took on a new and heightened urgency in these years.

Expectations surrounding female sexuality in the postwar years emphasized the importance of enjoyment and receptivity to sex but only within the confines of a very limiting ideal of heterosexual marriage. While the *Playboy* magazine issues of the period glorified exploitative escapades between married men and their unmarried secretaries, the wife at home was supposed to present dinner in high heels, pearls, and an alluring smile when her husband returned.[87] Female sexuality, unbounded, was particularly threatening during this period. As historian Elaine Tyler May argues in *Homeward Bound*, the containment of female sexuality safely within the bounds of heterosexual marriage and buried under the duties of housekeeping and motherhood served as a stabilizing social force throughout the Cold War era. Raising daughters in this context, mothers sought to nurture their girls' intelligent minds and emotional development, but only so they would be thoughtful and creative homemakers and mothers. As for their sexual development, girls needed to learn that their sexuality had to be contained, but not repressed, focused instead on the passive enjoyment of heterosexual sex some day with a husband.[88]

Much of the postwar era's advice to mothers on infant masturbation reads as a warning on how not to create "frigid" women during a time when medical experts on sex outlined carefully detailed theories about female sexual development. By the 1950s, as historian Carolyn Herbst Lewis has written, the medical community had thoroughly embraced Freudian ideas that the only psychologically normal sexual response in a properly matured woman was a vaginal orgasm.[89] Youthful clitoral pleasure, argued experts like psychiatrist Edward Bergler and gynecologist William S. Kroger, must shift to vaginal pleasure in adulthood in order for women to reach functional sexual maturity.[90] Historian Jessamyn Neuhaus has also observed a change in this period in the way marriage advice authors and psychiatrists thought and wrote about female sexuality and responsibility in marriage between the 1930s and 1950s, stating that by the postwar era, women who "experienced dissatisfaction" in their sex lives had only themselves to blame for refusing to "submit fully to [their] role as a wife and a mother."[91] The era's growing guidance around masturbation in female infants highlights that these broader cultural and medicalized ideas about gender, female sexual development, and dysfunction in the postwar years shaped the ways mothers and pediatricians thought about and addressed masturbation in young girls.

By the 1950s, mothers were learning to judge themselves based on their children's successful development into appropriately gendered, "functional" sexual adults, and pediatricians like Spock and those who had come before him had helped to establish that this work needed to begin soon after birth.[92] Spock styled himself actively as a "common sense" pediatrician, a phrase he adopted in the title of his famous childrearing manual. Thoroughly trained in both pediatric medicine and psychology, Spock helped translate and soften Freudian theories and behavioral research findings about childhood development for the masses in a way that many found reassuring. When it came to the highly charged issue of masturbation, it is no surprise that Spock found a way to explain what parents were seeing in a calm, nonthreatening, naturalistic way.

American children born since the 1950s have benefited from the move away from the era of mechanical restraints, surgical interventions, and drugs to combat self-pleasure, but anxieties and concerns about masturbation continued to linger through the end of the twentieth century, tied to tensions in broader cultural and medical ideas about sexuality and disguised in the rhetoric of "the natural."[93] In Spock's 1976 edition of his baby-rearing manual, "masturbation" once again appeared in the index, and it received a much lengthier treatment (perhaps in response to years of mothers' letters on the subject). Although he again assured his readers that bodily exploration is "wholesome curiosity" in infants, he provided updated information on children aged three to six that recalled the same anxieties and fears of earlier decades.[94] "We realize now that there is a childish kind of sexual feeling at this period, which is an essential part of normal development."[95] He continued, saying, "If you realize that this early interest in sex is a natural part of the slow process of growing up and that it occurs to a degree in all wholesome children, you can take a sensible view of it."[96] His discussion of this age group ended, nonetheless, with a jarring warning: "If a child is not preoccupied with sex, is generally outgoing, unworried, and has plenty of other interests and playmates, there is no cause for concern. If not, the child needs to be helped."[97] Although parents have repeatedly been told not to worry or overreact since the rise of "common sense" approaches to childcare, Spock's advice demonstrates that concerns about self-pleasure persisted despite the shift in rhetoric. Even Spock could not remove the sharp edge of worry and fear that masturbation, left unchecked, might cross the lines from "normal" to "abnormal" and harmless to harmful.

In writing to Spock, postwar mothers sought reassurance—were they handling their children's sexual development appropriately? Were they interfering too much? Too little? While they knew that their infants were not at risk of dire health outcomes from masturbation, mothers looked to their pediatricians for validation and help with the burden they carried: the task of raising children who could themselves reproduce their parents' middle-class life, built on the cornerstone of a sexually functional heterosexual marriage, with kids. By the 1950s, however, clinical pediatrics had largely turned its back on the issue of self-stimulation in very young children, leaving mothers with few places to turn for reassurance or advice. If a mother was able to solicit help from her pediatrician, by the end of the 1950s, these exchanges increasingly took the form of paternalistic condescension more than medical advice. Afterall, by the postwar years, being a good mother meant being in touch with one's "natural instinct" as much as it meant holding a rational appreciation for "natural" sexual behaviors, like masturbation in infancy.[98] As the pediatrician George H. Schade put it in 1958, "The management of [masturbation] in infancy requires a review of parental attitudes."[99] Caught between the expectations and demands of modern motherhood in the postwar years and the demedicalization of masturbatory behaviors in young children, mothers wrote worried letters and sent them off to experts like Spock, desperate to know if they were good mothers, capable of raising good boys and girls.

Notes

1. Letter to Spock (February 3, 1956), Group 1: Box 3, Folder: February 1956. Benjamin Spock and Mary Morgan Papers, Special Collections Research Center, Syracuse University Libraries.
2. Letter to Spock (February 3, 1956), Group 1: Box 3, Folder: February 1956.
3. Letter to Spock (March 18, 1957), Group 1: Box 3, Folder: March 1957.
4. E. Hare, "Masturbatory Insanity: The History of an Idea," *Journal of Mental Science* 108 (January 1962): 2–25; H. Tristram Engelhardt, "The Disease of Masturbation: Values and the Concept of Disease," *Bulletin of the History of Medicine* 48 (1974): 234–48; Michael Stolberg, "Self-Pollution, Moral Reform and the Venereal Trade: Notes on the Sources and Historical Context of Onania," *Journal of the History of Sexuality* 9 (2001): 37–61; Michael Stolberg, "An Unmanly Vice: Self-Pollution, Anxiety and the Body in the Eighteenth Century," *Social History of Medicine* 13 (2000): 1–21.
5. Rebecca Jo Plant, *Mom: The Transformation of American Motherhood* (Chicago: University of Chicago Press, 2010), 117. Plant writes extensively throughout this work about the tension in maternal expectations and roles during the mid-twentieth century. Her work highlights the impacts of an antimaternalism ideology that was particularly potent by the 1950s, one that portrayed mothers in a negative light while holding them almost exclusively responsible for the emotional and psychological health of their offspring.

6. Peter Gay, *Education of the Senses: The Bourgeois Experience—Victoria to Freud*, vol. 1 (New York: W. W. Norton & Company, 1984), 309; H. Tristram Englehardt Jr., "The Disease of Masturbation: Values and the Concept of Disease," in *Sickness and Health in America: Readings in the History of Medicine and Public Health*, ed. Judith Walzer Leavitt and Ronald L. Numbers, 2nd ed. (Madison: University of Wisconsin Press, 1985), 13; R. P. Newman, "Masturbation, Madness, and the Modern Concepts of Childhood and Adolescence," *Journal of Social History* 8 (1975): 1–2, 5.

7. Robert Darby, "A Post-Modernist Theory of Wanking," *Journal of Social History* 38, no. 1 (2004): 205–10.

8. Alan Hunt, "The Great Masturbation Panic and the Discourses of Moral Regulation in Nineteenth- and Early Twentieth-Century Britain," *Journal of the History of Sexuality* 8, no. 4 (1998): 575–615, 575.

9. Jean Stengers and Ann Van Neck, *Masturbation: The History of the Great Terror*, trans. Kathryn Hoffmann (New York: Palgrave, 2001).

10. R. P. Neuman, "Masturbation, Madness and the Modern Concepts of Childhood and Adolescence," *Journal of Social History* 8, no. 3 (1975): 1–27, see p. 14.

11. See, for example, Linda R. Watson, "The Universal Condition: Medical Constructions of 'Congenital Phimosis' in Twentieth Century New Zealand and Their Implications for Child Rearing," *Health and History* 16, no. 1 (2014): 87–106; Robert Darby, "Pathologizing Male Sexuality: Lallemand, Spermatorrhea, and the Rise of Circumcision," *Journal of the History of Medicine and Allied Sciences* 60, no. 3 (2005): 283–319; Robert Darby, "The Masturbation Taboo and the Rise of Routine Male Circumcision: A Review of the Historiography," *Journal of Social History* 36, no. 3 (2003): 737–57; Thomas Laqueur, *Solitary Sex: A Cultural History of Masturbation* (Brooklyn, NY: Zone Books, 2003); James R. Kincaid, "What the Victorians Knew about Sex," *Browning Institute Studies* 16 (1988): 91–99.

12. See, for example, Joan Jacobs Brumberg, *The Body Project: An Intimate History of American Girls* (New York: Vintage, 1998), 160–65, 173; Rachel P. Maines, *The Technology of Orgasm: "Hysteria," the Vibrator, and Women's Sexual Satisfaction* (Baltimore: Johns Hopkins University Press, 1999), 56–59; Andrew Scull, *Hysteria: The Disturbing History* (Oxford: Oxford University Press, 2012), 74–79.

13. Lesley A. Hall, "Forbidden by God, Despised by Men: Masturbation, Medical Warnings, Moral Panic, and Manhood in Great Britain, 1850–1950," *Journal of the History of Sexuality* 2, no. 3 (1992): 365–87, see p. 372.

14. Neuman, "Masturbation, Madness and the Modern Concepts of Childhood and Adolescence," especially 13–16.

15. Michael S. Patton, "Twentieth-Century Attitudes Toward Masturbation," *Journal of Religion and Health* 25, no. 4 (1986): 291–302.

16. Alfred C. Kinsey, Wardell B. Pomeroy, and Clyde E. Martin, *Sexual Behavior in the Human Male* (Philadelphia: W. B. Saunders, 1948); Alfred C. Kinsey, Clyde E. Martin, Paul H. Gebhard, Wardell Baxter Pomeroy, George Washington Corner, and Robert M. Yerkes, *Sexual Behavior in the Human Female* (Philadelphia: W. B. Saunders, 1953).

17. Nancy Pottishman Weiss first noted this phenomenon in child/mother dynamics in her 1977 analysis of midcentury childrearing manuals. See Weiss, "Mother, the Invention of Necessity: Dr. Benjamin Spock's Baby and Child Care," *American Quarterly* 29, no. 5 (Winter 1977): 519–46, see p. 533. See also Michale A. Sulman, "The Humanization of the American Child: Benjamin Spock as a Popularizer of Psychoanalytic Thought," *Journal of the History of the Behavioral Sciences* 9, no. 3 (1973): 258–65;

Julia Grant, *Raising Baby by the Book: The Education of American Mothers* (New Haven, CT: Yale University Press, 1998); Anne Hulbert, *Raising America: Experts, Parents, and a Century of Advice about Children* (New York: Knopf, 2003).

18. Alfred Vogel, *A Practical Treatise on the Diseases of Children*, trans. Henry Raphael (New York: Appleton, 1870), 461.

19. Vogel as quoted in Milton I. Levine and Anita I. Bell, "The Psychologic Aspects of Pediatric Practice: II. Masturbation," *Pediatrics* 18, no. 5 (1956): 803–8.

20. L. Emmett Holt, *The Diseases of Infancy and Childhood: For the Use of Students and Practitioners of Medicine* (New York: Appleton, 1897), 696–97.

21. Holt (1897), 696–97.

22. Holt (1897), 696–97.

23. L. Emmett Holt, *The Diseases of Infancy and Childhood: For the Use of Students and Practitioners of Medicine*, 5th ed. (New York, Appleton, 1909), 744–45.

24. Holt (1897), 697.

25. Holt (1897), 698.

26. Holt (1909), 746. For more on the history of female circumcision as a medical treatment for sexual pathology in Western societies, see Sarah W. Rodriguez, "Rethinking the History of Female Circumcision and Clitoridectomy: American Medicine and Female Sexuality in the Late Nineteenth Century," *Journal of the History of Medicine and Allied Sciences* 63, no. 3 (July 2008): 323–47.

27. Holt (1909), 744.

28. Holt (1909), 746.

29. Holt (1909), 746.

30. Work done on the history of medical circumcision in New Zealand in the first half of the twentieth century, for example, has demonstrated that Holt's suggested link between masturbation in male infants and irritation supposedly caused by an attached foreskin appeared in parent advice and medical literature throughout midcentury, helping to eventually universalize male circumcision in infants there after World War I. See Lindsay R. Watson, "The Universal Condition: Medical Constructions of 'Congenital Phimosis' in Twentieth Century New Zealand and Their Implications for Child Rearing," *Health and History* 16, no. 1 (2014): 87–106.

31. Discussion in Levine and Bell, "The Psychologic Aspects of Pediatric Practice."

32. Janet Golden, *Babies Made Us Modern: How Infants Brought America into the Twentieth Century* (Cambridge: Cambridge University Press, 2018), 141–65.

33. Kathleen W. Jones, "Sentiment and Science: The Late Nineteenth Century Pediatrician as Mother's Advisor," *Journal of Social History* 17, no. 1 (1983): 79–96, quote on p. 80.

34. Elisha Mather Sill, *The Child: Its Care, Diet and Common Ills* (New York: Henry Holt and Company, 1913), 153.

35. Cornell University, *The Register, 1904–1905* (Ithaca, NY: Cornell University, 1905), 227; Thomas William Herringshaw, *The American Physician and Surgeon Blue Book: A Distinct Cyclopedia of 1919* (Chicago: American Blue Book Publishers, 1919), 400.

36. Sill, *The Child*, 153.

37. Sill, 153.

38. Sill, 154.

39. Sill, 154.

40. Sill, 154.

41. Mary Mills West, *Infant Care*, rev. ed. (Washington, D.C.: Government Printing Office, 1922 [reprint of the 1921 edition]), 45–46. Historian Molly Ladd-Taylor discusses the

shifts in tone and authorship in the Children's Bureau's *Infant Care* pamphlets, noting that the 1914 and 1921 editions were both written by West. By the 1929 revision, authored by Dr. Martha Eliot, the Children's Bureau's willingness to dispense health-related advice had waned. By the end of the 1920s, the medically controlled department's standard response to mothers' letters became "consult a physician." See Molly Ladd-Taylor, *Raising a Baby the Government Way: Mothers' Letters to the Children's Bureau, 1915–1932* (New Brunswick, NJ: Rutgers University Press, 1986), 23.

42. Emily K. Abel, "Benevolence and Social Control: Advice from the Children's Bureau in the Early Twentieth Century," *Social Service Review* 68, no. 1 (1994): 1–19, p. 4.

43. Ladd-Taylor, *Raising a Baby*, 44.

44. West, *Infant Care* (1922), 46.

45. West, 46.

46. West, 46.

47. Carolyn Conant Van Blarcom, *Building the Baby: The Foundation for Robust and Efficient Men and Women* (Chicago: Chicago Tribute, 1929), 89.

48. Van Blarcom, 89.

49. Van Blarcom, 89.

50. Neuman, "Masturbation, Madness and the Modern Concepts of Childhood and Adolescence," 16.

51. Ruth Morris Bakwin and Harry Bakwin, *Psychologic Care during Infancy and Childhood* (New York: D. Appleton, 1942), 265–66.

52. Bakwin and Bakwin, 266.

53. Deborah Blythe Doroshow, "An Alarming Solution: Bedwetting, Medicine, and Behavioral Conditioning in Mid-Twentieth-Century America," *Isis* 101, no. 2 (2010): 312–37.

54. Bakwin and Bakwin, *Psychologic Care*, 265.

55. Bakwin and Bakwin, 266.

56. Bakwin and Bakwin, 266.

57. Benjamin Spock, *Common Sense Book of Baby and Child Care* (New York: Duell, Sloan and Pearce, 1946), 300.

58. Spock, 300.

59. Spock, 300.

60. Spock, 300.

61. Spock, 300.

62. Spock, 301.

63. Spock, 303.

64. Spock, 303.

65. Grant, *Raising Baby*, 161.

66. In 1947, St. Joseph Aspirin for Children hit the market, providing pediatricians and parents with access to a candy-flavored, over-the-counter medication that spurred use of the medicine for all manner of childhood discomforts. See Cynthia A. Connolly, *Balancing Risk and Prevention in Twentieth-Century America* (New Brunswick, NJ: Rutgers University Press, 2018), 96–102.

67. Levine and Bell, "The Psychologic Aspects of Pediatric Practice," 804.

68. Levine and Bell, 804.

69. Grant, *Raising Baby*, 161.

70. Laqueur, *Solitary Sex*, 359.

71. Grant, *Raising Baby*, 161.

72. Grant writes at length about how mothers actually viewed or utilized expert childrearing advice. Grant, *Raising Baby*, 138.

73. Grant, *Raising Baby*, 216.

74. Nicola Kay Beisel, *Imperiled Innocents, Anthony Comstock and Family Reproduction in Victorian America* (Princeton, NJ: Princeton University Press, 1997), 2–5.

75. Neuman, "Masturbation, Madness and the Modern Concepts of Childhood and Adolescence."

76. Elaine Tyler May, *Homeward Bound: American Families in the Cold War Era* (New York: Basic Books, 2008), 162–68.

77. Peter N. Stearns, *Anxious Parents: A History of Modern Childrearing in America* (New York: New York University Press, 2003), 108–9.

78. See, for example Niles R. Newton, *The Family Book of Childcare* (New York, NY: Harper Press, 1957), 290–303.

79. Influential child development and culture experts such as Margaret Ribble, Margaret Mead, and Niles Newton, for example, alongside the tremendously well-known Benjamin Spock, helped popularize a more palatable interpretation of Freudian sexual development for parents. Rather than suppressing natural urges, this strain of thought emphasized the importance of ushering children through critical periods of development unscathed. Negative interference in this "natural" developmental arc could arrest development or divert it, harming the child's potential to grow into a heterosexual adult. See Jessica Martucci, *Back to the Breast: Natural Motherhood and Breastfeeding in America* (Chicago: University of Chicago Press, 2015), 45–57. See also Henry Jenkins, "The Sensuous Child: Dr. Benjamin Spock and the Sexual Revolution," in *The Children's Culture Reader*, edited by Henry Jenkins (New York: New York University Press, 1998), 209–30.

80. Historian Rebecca Jo Plant's work on important shifts in American motherhood during the mid-twentieth century is extremely enlightening and essential reading for anyone interested in the history of parenting, women, childhood, or the family. Rebecca Jo Plant, *Mom: The Transformation of Motherhood in Modern America* (Chicago: University of Chicago Press, 2010), 45–54.

81. Donna Penn, "The Meanings of Lesbianism in Post-War America," *Gender & History* 3, no. 2 (1991): 190–203.

82. Margot Canaday, *The Straight State: Sexuality and Citizenship in Twentieth-Century America* (Princeton, NJ: Princeton University Press, 2009), 4–5.

83. Plant, *Mom*, 104–6.

84. Peter Stearns, "Historical Perspectives on Twentieth-Century American Childhood," in *Beyond the Century of the Child: Cultural History and Developmental Psychology*, ed. Willem Koops and Michael Zuckerman (Philadelphia: University of Pennsylvania Press, 2003), 96–111, p. 101.

85. Letter to Spock (August 21, 1959), Group 1: Box 5, Folder: August 1959.

86. For example, see Carol Groneman, "Nymphomania: The Historical Construction of Female Sexuality," *Signs* 19, no. 2 (1994): 337–67. Also, Molly Ladd-Taylor discusses the intersection in twentieth-century eugenic laws over labels of "feeble-mindedness" and charges of "promiscuity" or any sexual behavior outside of marriage. See Molly Ladd-Taylor, *Fixing the Poor: Eugenic Sterilization and Child Welfare in the Twentieth Century* (Baltimore: Johns Hopkins University Press, 2017).

87. Based on my review of issues of *Playboy* magazines from its first issue in December 1953 through December 1968 from the microfilm collections of Van Pelt Library at the University of Pennsylvania.

88. Elaine Tyler May, *Homeward Bound: American Families in the Cold War Era*, rev. ed. (New York: Basic Books, 2017).

89. Carolyn Herbst Lewis, *Prescription for Heterosexuality: Sexual Citizenship in the Cold War Era* (Chapel Hill: University of North Carolina Press, 2010), 37–70.

90. Lewis, 40.

91. Jessamyn Neuhaus, "The Importance of Being Orgasmic: Sexuality, Gender, and Marital Sex Manuals in the United States, 1920–1963," *Journal of the History of Sexuality*, 9, no. 4 (2000): 447–73, see p. 461.

92. Jenkins, "The Sensuous Child," 209–30.

93. For more on the role of nature ideology in late twentieth-century parenting and pediatrics, see Martucci, *Back to the Breast*.

94. Benjamin Spock, *Baby and Child Care* (New York: Hawthorn Books,1976), 387.

95. Spock, 387.

96. Spock, 387.

97. Spock, 387.

98. Grant, *Raising Baby*, 209–11.

99. George H. Schade, "Masturbation in Children," *Pediatric Clinics of North America* 5, no. 3 (1958): 767–74, p. 768.

Chapter 3

Gender and Doctor–Parent Communication about Down Syndrome in the Mid-Twentieth Century

HUGHES EVANS

In 1944, child development expert Erik Erikson's wife and collaborator, Joan, gave birth to a son, Neil. Several days later, Erikson went home and told his children that Neil had died and that the family should not discuss the topic. Actually, Neil was not dead but had been diagnosed with Mongolism (today known as Down syndrome). Their doctors informed Erikson that Neil would not live more than a year or two and recommended immediate institutionalization. While Joan was under anesthesia, Erikson reached out to two close friends for advice, anthropologist Margaret Mead and Jungian analyst Joseph Wheelwright. Mead strongly agreed with the doctors, warning that a disabled child would disrupt their household and stating that institutionalization was best for both Neil and the family. Mead also advised Erikson to prevent Joan from seeing or holding her son, saying that to do so would only make it more difficult for her to give him up. Erikson decided to institutionalize his son without consulting with his wife.[1] Neil lived the next twenty-one years in an institution.[2]

Twenty-two years later, in 1966, playwright Arthur Miller's third wife, Inge Morath, gave birth to a son with Down syndrome, Daniel. Like Neil, Daniel entered an institution shortly after birth, and, like Erikson, Miller did not discuss his son publicly. Friends recalled that Inge wanted to keep Daniel but that Arthur would not allow it, that he worried that raising Daniel would be difficult for their daughter and their household.[3] Miller reflected on Daniel's birth in a 1968 journal entry, saying, "As the nurse was dressing Daniel in the hospital, preparing him for our journey to the institution, I turned to examine him—with some difficulty. In a few seconds I found myself, not doubting the doctor's conclusions, but feeling a welling up of love for him. I dared not touch him, lest I end up taking him home, and I wept."[4] Although Inge visited her son in the facility, Miller never did. Miller did, however, remember Daniel in his will, granting him an equal share of his estate. Reflecting on her parents' actions, Daniel's older sister Rebecca felt they would have said "that they were advised to do it. That he believed that it was the right thing for our family. It's a subject that was just hard to broach in my family. And when you're raised like that, it's not easy to just overcome that right away."[5]

During the middle decades of the twentieth century, physicians overwhelmingly advised parents of newborns with Down syndrome to place their babies as soon as possible in residential facilities for the "mentally retarded." The advice to institutionalize was not limited to Down syndrome; children with many other forms of mental and developmental delay also tended to enter facilities (albeit later). Down syndrome was unique. A relatively common condition (it occurred in 1 of every 500–700 births), it composed the most frequent congenital cause of intellectual delay. What's more, doctors could easily recognize the distinctive features shortly after birth—long before most other causes of intellectual impairment became apparent. While other causes of so-called retardation became gradually evident as parents noticed that their child could not keep up with other children his or her age, the intellectual challenges of the child with Down syndrome could be predicted from early infancy. As Dr. Alfred Franklin, a London pediatrician, noted, "What singles out this problem is, first, that it concerns mental defect, and, secondly, . . . the first look at the head and face, before the whole baby is born, can reveal diagnosis and prognosis, the sadder because medicine cannot help."[6] Most experts agreed that over 90 percent of babies with Down syndrome could be diagnosed at birth or shortly thereafter.[7] The fact that it could be diagnosed so early precipitated a "crisis"—an urgent and immediate decision for parents who had just met their baby.[8]

Both Erikson and Miller were famous; their stories, however, were commonplace. Through a twenty-first-century lens, their actions appear inhumane, but when placed in the context of the mid-twentieth century, decisions such as theirs reflect the prevailing mores, professional values, and notions of family and gender. Nevertheless, these stories are striking for many reasons. They imply commonly held beliefs about Down syndrome as a feared and stigmatized condition with fixed expectations about ultimate development and life span. Equally impressive are the similarities in how both husbands made their decision to institutionalize their sons, with little to no input from their wives, relying on physicians trained to provide authoritarian and paternalistic advice. Deeply ingrained medical and professional roles shaped the decision-making process in terms of who was informed, when they were told, how the conversation unfolded, and the ultimate decision to institutionalize. This chapter examines this critical diagnostic and therapeutic moment through the lens of changing gender norms in the mid-twentieth century.

In the middle of the twentieth century, Down syndrome was referred to as "mongoloid idiocy," a term coined by John Langdon Down in 1866.[9] At the time, Down worked as the medical superintendent at the Royal Earlswood Asylum for Idiots in Sussex, England.[10] He noticed that a subset of the Earlswood residents had similar physical features and proposed that they constituted a unique syndrome of intellectual delay. Down believed that the defining characteristics represented a throwback to an earlier, primitive, what he termed "Mongol" type.[11] Although the scientific community subsequently rejected Down's racial atavism theory, the name mongolism and its variations stuck well into the 1970s.[12]

Over the decades following Down's initial description, some took issue with the name and its misleading reference to Mongolia and offered other monikers. Clemens E. Benda, MD, a leading Down syndrome researcher and physician at the Wrentham State School for the Feebleminded in Wrentham, Massachusetts, urged the adoption of Lionel Penrose's suggestion, congenital acromicria. This name referred to the typically small hands and feet in Down syndrome, but the designation never stuck.[13] After French scientist Jerome Lejeune discovered the chromosomal basis of Down syndrome in 1959 (the extra chromosome 21), the term "trisomy 21" began to circulate, but it, too, did not take hold outside of scientific circles. Two years later, in 1961, prominent scientists and physicians published a letter in The Lancet urging the medical and scientific community to abandon the term "mongolism."[14] The World Health Organization officially discarded the term "mongolism" in 1966 after a delegation from The People's Republic of Mongolian objected to its use.[15] Despite these official changes, the terms "mongol" and "mongolism" continued to be commonly used by experts as well as the lay public.

Mongolism and its derivations acquired negative connotations, in part because any word denoting intellectual delay hinted at eugenic beliefs that "feeblemindedness" ran in families. Popularized in the early twentieth century, eugenics warned that mental impairments represented a familial genetic stain.[16] In addition, eugenics taught that mental impairment went hand in hand with undesirable characteristics such as sexual promiscuity and criminality, further marring an already stigmatized condition. New parents worried that a mentally disabled child would cast a shadow over their entire family and mark them with undesirable, even criminal characteristics. Parents worried that a mentally impaired child would ruin the chances of their other children—especially their daughters—to date and marry. Even though Down syndrome was not inherited, it acquired a similar stigma. Because Down syndrome could be diagnosed so early in life, families were forced to address the eugenic implications earlier than with other causes of mental delay. After the birth of a child with Down syndrome, the lens of eugenics cast doubts on the inherent social value of the parents; the mother's reproductive and caregiving role was blemished and the father's provider role was equally tarnished.

Even after eugenics had been debunked, the diagnosis of Down syndrome continued to be discussed in hushed tones and had an undeniable impact on common perceptions of mental disability.[17] As a 1945 *Saturday Evening Post* article noted,

> Chances are high that you never heard of the condition called "Mongolism." In a needlessly sinister context, however, it may have shown itself among your acquaintances. Neighbors of yours, you remember, were finally expecting a baby and, having waited long for it, were heartwarmingly delighted. The approximate due date arrived, but you heard nothing more—or maybe too much. There were whispers that the child was "queer"; that the Neighbors had to have it sent away; that it was a terrible thing, and Mr. and Mrs. Neighbor had always seemed like such nice normal people. Nobody was very specific, but it was plain that something horrible had happened and that even mentioning parenthood in the Neighbors presence would be utterly unkind. That may well have been a Mongoloid child, a poor little stunted thing doomed to lag forever far below normal development of physique, intellect and emotions.[18]

Doctors, especially pediatricians, played a key role shaping the perception of Down syndrome. The specialty had been established in the late nineteenth century, but few physicians limited their practice to children until the mid-twentieth century.[19] The rise of "scientific motherhood" in the early twentieth century, with its reliance on the pediatrician as an authority concerning all issues related to child health and disease, made the pediatrician the expert.[20] With a plethora of babies to care for in the postwar years, pediatricians busily developed therapies for diseases that previously had stymied efforts. Advances in nutrition, vaccines, and especially antibiotics yielded impressive results. The infant mortality rate plummeted and life expectancy rose.[21] Pediatricians wrote columns in popular ladies' magazines and authored popular child care books.[22] Benjamin Spock's bestselling *Common Sense Book of Baby and Child Care* epitomized the pediatrician as childcare expert—including numerous editions and selling over 24 million copies by 1972.[23] In the paternalistic mode typical of early twentieth-century medicine, doctors, including pediatricians, frequently told patients, or parents, what to do, rather than advised them. While impressive strides were made treating infectious diseases, endocrine disorders, and causes of malnutrition, the diseases causing intellectual impairment proved more difficult to address.

The so-called mental retardation diseases saw some diagnostic breakthroughs in the first half of the twentieth century, but therapies were elusive until several decades later. For instance, patients with hypothyroidism, or cretinism, as it was commonly called at the time, received thyroid hormone with impressive results starting in the 1890s, but the brain damage from congenital hypothyroidism was typically irreversible before clinical signs showed themselves. Therefore, while thyroid hormone therapy generated enthusiasm, it was not until the advent of newborn screening in the 1970s that the therapy yielded neurodevelopmental results.[24] Similarly, during the early 1940s, scientists recognized that German measles caused congenital rubella syndrome—a constellation of features that included blindness, heart disease, hearing impairment, and mental delay.[25] While there was no treatment for congenital rubella once it had occurred, a vaccine became widely available in 1969 and led to many fewer cases.[26] Dietary treatment for phenylketonuria, a rare genetic cause of intellectual delay, slowed or stopped progression of the disease but required widespread newborn screening to identify the affected infants.[27] Research on these conditions contributed to a mood of optimism regarding the eventual ability of biomedicine to make significant breakthroughs in the previously impervious causes of childhood intellectual delay, but efforts to find a viable treatment for Down syndrome proved fruitless. Some scientists touted surgical treatments or medical regimens with glutamic acid and various hormone extracts, but nothing worked, and many worried that these therapies had led parents on a wild goose chase for an elusive cure. The lack of progress in the search for a viable Down syndrome treatment contributed to a general belief that Down syndrome was "hopeless."[28] Frustrated by the lack of meaningful treatment, primary care physicians as well as specialists framed the diagnosis as a lost cause and disparaged parents' fruitless searches for a cure.[29]

In these postwar years, the ideal family was happy, healthy, and wholesome.[30] The middle and upper classes were overwhelmingly Caucasian and upwardly mobile. Little room existed for a child with mental delay. What's more, traditional gender roles for mothers and fathers reinforced the expectation of a brood of "normal" children.[31] Mothers were judged by the quality of their children and the homes they kept, while fathers were measured by their ability to provide

for their families. Education and intellectual attainment were paths to social success. Children became visible indicators of parental achievement. In this era,
the popularization of Freudian thought frequently cast blame on mothers for
their children's problems.[32] Women who were emotionally distant—the so-
called refrigerator mothers—were implicated for causing autism in their children.[33] The overprotective mother, on the other hand, might smother her children
and prevent them from developing properly.

Children who did not fit this happy mold represented failure, and parents
suffered under the stigma entailed by mental retardation in general and Down
syndrome in particular. Reports abounded that children with intellectual delay
were sequestered in their homes, their families fearful of what neighbors would
say and think. Dr. Fanny Stang warned of the danger of parents "shutting themselves away with their defective child like lepers."[34] Physicians endeavored to
explain to parents that Down syndrome was not inherited, but the pervasive bias
proved insidious and difficult for many families to overcome. Dr. Harry Goldstein, writing in 1954, urged fellow physicians to "encourage the mentally
retarded children's parents not to be ashamed to take their children to places of
interest, and to visit friends and family. Parents must not keep the children
parked in their homes, and shut out from the rest of the world."[35] Despite Goldstein's advice to his colleagues, many physicians shared societal concerns about
Down syndrome and urged anxious parents to institutionalize their babies.

While not all doctors agreed that institutionalization was best, most followed the advice promoted by prominent pediatricians in textbooks and journals. Some pediatricians traced the efforts to institutionalize in infancy to Joseph
Brennemann, a leading pediatrician in Chicago and later Los Angeles, and
author of a major pediatrics textbook that went through numerous editions. They
claimed that Brennemann held that the pediatrician should "practically . . .
demand that the mother should not take the child home from the hospital with
her but should place it immediately in an institution."[36] Another prominent
pediatrician in this camp was the Mayo Clinic's C. Anderson Aldrich. Known
for championing infants as individuals, Dr. Aldrich coauthored a popular childrearing book with his wife, entitled *Babies Are Human Beings: An Interpretation of Growth*.[37] The book celebrated early childhood development and the role
of the child in the family but ignored babies with developmental delays. Starting in the 1930s, Aldrich began promoting his method for convincing parents
to commit newborns with Down syndrome. The stakes were high for these families. If parents did not follow his advice, he warned, the mother would become
"a complete slave to his dependency" and subsequently neglect her household
duties, her other children, and her husband.[38] The siblings would feel so

ashamed that they would "refuse to bring other children into the house."[39] Marital relations would deteriorate, and divorce would ensue. Aldrich elaborated his technique "to lessen all this grief."[40] Key to his method's success was separating the baby from the mother and preventing mother–infant bonding, made possible, he believed, because doctors could diagnose Down syndrome at birth in more than 90 percent of cases. He outlined four steps:[41]

1. First, after birth, tell the mother that the baby "is not strong enough" and "must remain in the nursery."
2. Second, meet immediately with the father and close relatives and outline the nature of the diagnosis, its seriousness, that no one is to blame, that future babies will be normal, and that "immediate placement outside the family provides the only hope of preventing a long series of family difficulties."
3. Third, after convincing the father of the benefits of outside placement, then inform the mother that the doctor, father, and relatives have made the decision. In other words, "She is asked, not to *make* the decision, but to accept the one which has already been made by the close relatives."
4. Finally, the physician arranges for immediate placement in an institution or a boarding home.

Aldrich's plan placed the decision to institutionalize firmly on male shoulders. The job of the physician (who was almost always a man) was to convince the family of the proper course of action. The strategy relied on time-honored beliefs that men were more practical, were better able to make sound decisions, and had the emotional fortitude to handle what was commonly considered a family tragedy. Aldrich's approach depended on overruling any strong emotional beliefs the mother might have and relied on convincing the father that this was the best course of action. By drawing on commonly held masculine traits, the doctor could forge an alliance with the father and convince him of the best course of action.[42] Together they would enlist additional support from the family, and the entire group would, in essence, overrule any contrary opinions that the mother may have. The goal was to remove the mother's agency and decision-making capacity. Aldrich, and many like him, framed the child with Down syndrome as a "threat to the continual well-being of family life."[43]

According to Dr. Arthur Parmelee, many pediatricians followed Aldrich's method "enthusiastically and . . . almost fanatically."[44] Experts at Washington's Children's Hospital estimated that 80 percent of pediatricians recommended institutionalization at birth.[45] Others placed this number even higher.[46] Numerous doctors elaborated on Aldrich's method, drawing on their own experience. Dr. John Washington advised, "When the diagnosis is made in the nursery it is well to stay away from the mother's room until arrangements can be made to have the father and, if possible, the obstetrician present. In ordinary circumstances it is not fair to the mother to withhold the truth; on the other hand, she should not be faced with such disturbing news unsupported by her family and medical aid. Calling the obstetrician is the first move, after which the father should be contacted and informed of the true situation."[47] Another doctor agreed, saying, "It's better to institutionalize early. The longer it takes, the longer 'the knife is in the side.'"[48] One survey of parents who committed their children revealed that 91 percent did so because of their physician's encouragement.[49] Aldrich's method offered a path through a thorny problem for doctors and parents.

Aldrich and others believed this approach was possible because they could prevent or minimize the mother's interaction with her baby. Some recommended thwarting opportunities for the mother to see or hold her baby. Others were more specific and discouraged interactions that promoted bonding, such as breast-feeding.[50] Citing the need to protect the wife from her maternal instinct to care for her baby, some doctors occasionally colluded with fathers in lying to mothers that the baby had died.[51] One father, who was pressured to arrange immediate admission to a facility so that his wife could be told that the child had died, asked, "How can I live with my wife and live with such a lie?"[52] Such subterfuge was impossible in some situations, but numerous stories existed of siblings and neighbors learning years later that the supposedly dead child actually resided in an institution.[53] A number of doctors, however, were uncomfortable with this ploy, calling it both practically difficult and morally repugnant. Others pointed to the impossibility of preventing bonding, saying it had already occurred during pregnancy.[54]

Informing the father first about the suspected diagnosis appeared to come naturally to many physicians. Fathers awaited news about the birth in the hospital waiting room, and doctors commonly updated fathers after a delivery.[55] Male doctors may have felt more comfortable sharing such difficult news with another man. Midcentury medicine was steeped in paternalism; important conversations naturally occurred man to man. Doctors expressed concern regarding the emotional impact on the mother, and many hoped to avoid such an uncomfortable conversation. Fathers were further removed from the emotional center of the home and thus able to think dispassionately about the situation or even to deny the impact. Noted psychiatrist Leo Kanner elaborated on paternal denial, a common reaction to a child's mental delay diagnosis, saying, "This is often the reaction especially of fathers who have no knowledge of children and do not wish to be bothered about them. They are away at work most of the day, have a glimpse of the child when he is asleep, hear the child's laughter on the rare occasion when they pick him up, and conclude with a shrug of the shoulder: 'I can't see anything unusual.'"[56] Some doctors asked the husband to tell his wife the diagnosis, arguing that it would soften the blow. Others would inform a father shortly after birth and advise him to hold off telling his wife until the diagnosis was confirmed or a plan was in place. Some even urged that the gentlest method was to let the mother figure it out on her own. This rationale insinuated that the mother was a simpleton herself, unable to appreciate the fact that her baby looked different, was floppier than other babies, and did not develop at the same rate. British psychologist Janet Carr followed a cohort of parents and their children with Down syndrome for many years and disagreed with encouraging fathers to withhold the diagnosis from their wives. "This seems too heavy a burden to impose, and one that a father should not be expected to bear, or anyway not for longer than a day or two," she argued.[57] Psychiatrist Valerie Cowie offered a very practical reason to inform the father first that hinted at the lingering stigma surrounding the diagnosis. "It would seem to be kinder to tell the father as soon as the diagnosis is firmly made," she stated. "The announcement in the 'Births' column of a newspaper might be phrased differently if the father knew he was announcing to the world the birth of a mongol."[58]

Many opted for the Aldrich method to tell the father first, formulate a plan, and then inform the mother. A survey of thirty-five Washington, D.C. physicians in 1961 reported that approximately twenty-two spoke to fathers first, ten notified both parents together, and only two told the mother first.[59] Doctors rationalized apprising the father first with explanations that reflected widely held beliefs about women's emotional fragility and the father's role as head of the household. These clinicians warned that the postpartum emotional rollercoaster rendered a mother incapable of making important decisions regarding her baby and suggested waiting at least four to six weeks to tell her the diagnosis.[60] Even a mother, speaking at a 1960 conference in Glasgow, agreed with waiting to divulge the diagnosis, saying that "many mothers in the days immediately following the birth may be considered not to be stable."[61] Journalist Ridgely Hunt wrote about this issue several years later in a 1967 *Chicago Tribune* exposé on children with Down syndrome entitled "The Unfinished Children." In it, Hunt warned about the problems that the parents must face, saying, "The first, and in some respects the most difficult, problem concerns the mother. She has just suffered the ordeal of childbirth. Her body aches, her stomach is upset, her hormones and emotions are badly out of balance. Her one consolation in this hour of physical and psychological exhaustion is the presence of her baby, whose advent she has anticipated with pleasure for nine months. And now the baby is broken. He may not survive infancy, and even if he does, he will never have a normal body or a normal mind."[62]

Doctors' rationales about when to divulge the diagnosis also reflected a number of common concerns regarding medical confirmation of the diagnosis, the doctors' own feelings about Down syndrome, and the implications for the parents. Some worried about inflicting damage and heartache with a mistaken diagnosis and urged caution in mentioning their suspicions until receiving a second opinion. As more doctors chose to specialize in pediatrics, general practitioners and obstetricians, who had previously been the first doctors to recognize the problem, turned to child specialists, both to confirm the suspected bad news and increasingly to find a "child specialist" to conduct the difficult conversation. Before the discovery of trisomy 21, the diagnosis relied on telltale physical exam findings. During the 1960s, doctors began to submit genetic testing, a process that could take several excruciating weeks. Some physicians appeared to take a path of avoidance in which one or both parents would come to the realization of their child's limitations on their own. While some professionals felt such an approach was gentle, others felt this represented "a reluctance on the part of physicians to deal with the emotional reactions of both parents at the same time."[63] Two experts on mental retardation, commenting on delays in diagnosis, pointed out that the "physician often faces crises within himself."[64] These perspectives suggested a physician might not tell a parent the diagnosis or might delay "because of his past experiences with retarded children, his attitudes towards social incompetency, his difficulty in making value judgments, the parents' questions, etc."[65] These physicians, they said, "may resort to defensive mechanisms, such as avoiding the diagnosis, reassuring the parents, making dogmatic statements, e.g., a 'mongoloid child should not be seen by the mother,' etc."[66]

Conditions associated with Down syndrome further complicated the picture. Doctors knew that some, but not all, affected infants suffered from varying degrees of heart and gastrointestinal defects. Duodenal atresia, for instance, was a deadly complication until surgical correction became increasingly available in the 1950s. At the time, many physicians felt conflicted about whether to fix these life-threatening abnormalities in a child diagnosed with "mongolism," and parents were similarly ambivalent about the ultimate utility of surgical correction in their child.[67] These newborns were often moved to the back of the nursery, where they eventually died of starvation or other causes.[68] Doctors rarely discussed withholding lifesaving treatment from Down syndrome newborns in the midcentury medical literature, yet the practice was relatively common. While clearly morally distressing for all involved, the unspoken agreement about the futility of surgery for these children further underscores the pervasiveness of the stigma around Down syndrome and the paternalism of the medical profession.

Not all physicians agreed with Aldrich and adopted his plan. Arthur Parmelee found it "morally and ethically unsound."[69] Doctors affiliated with institutions expressed particular concern about separating newborn children from their families. Two superintendents at Canadian facilities took strong issue, arguing that institutionalization amounted to "disposal of the mongol child" and denied mothers their "right to mourn."[70] Pediatrician and psychiatrist Donald Jolly claimed in 1953 that placing infants in chronic care facilities had been a rising trend since the late 1930s and had reached an "extreme situation" with mongolism.[71] A medical superintendent at the Wrentham State School, Jolly had firsthand knowledge of the clamor to institutionalize newborns and opposed the practice. He disagreed with the rationale that preventing mother–infant bonding led to better outcomes. "In most cases the mother is already attached to the child," he cautioned. "Her attachment has literally and figuratively grown during pregnancy." Jolly provided an example describing a mother of an infant with Down syndrome whose husband prevented her from seeing the baby and arranged immediate institutionalization. "Broken up over the whole thing," the mother suffered considerably. Her husband eventually relented and allowed her to see their critically ill baby. "Why, she's not so bad," said the mother, who then "broke down, and enjoyed a much needed cry."[72] Wishing to avoid this type of heartache, Jolly advocated to send the affected baby home, where the mother would gradually become aware of its deficiencies and ultimately recognize institutionalization as the best option. He urged placement after age three.[73] Jolly's parable reflected ways in which management of an infant with Down syndrome embraced firmly entrenched gender stereotypes. He noted that a decision to immediately transfer the neonate from hospital nursery to an institution might be "the simplest one for the physician" but was "seldom the best solution for the parents and other members of the family."[74]

Physicians warned parents that implications of the diagnosis extended beyond the child to affect the entire family. As one physician remarked, "It is true that mongolism is primarily a family problem."[75] Doctors urged parents to consider the repercussions on their other children, and parents took this advice to heart. Richard Tudor, a Minneapolis pediatrician, felt the potential untoward consequences on siblings were often the "deciding factor" in decisions to institutionalize.[76] Doctors warned that the diagnosis would cast a pall over an entire family and that the siblings would feel the stigma disproportionately. "Normal" siblings would be embarrassed by their affected sibling and hesitate to bring friends home, leading to social isolation for the children. Perhaps most worrisome was the potential impact on able-bodied girls as they approached the age to date and marry. Parents were particularly concerned that the eugenic stain of the diagnosis would ward off potential suitors from courting their daughters. One father of a child with Down syndrome reared at home complained, "My daughter should be thinking of marriage. What chance does she have? Her life is being ruined."[77]

The concerns about the effect on siblings often revolved around the mother's ability to fulfill her maternal duties. The so-called retarded child would usurp so much of her energy that she would not have the time or emotional energy for her other children. The "normal" children would feel neglected and suffer from this deprivation of maternal love. These arguments often drove at the core of parental worries about providing the best possible home for their family. No parent wanted to inadvertently hurt one of their children because they were caring for a child with Down syndrome. As journalist Ridgely Hunt explained, "The mother may fear that, in caring for the mongoloid, she will neglect her other children, making them hostile and resentful. Often, too, she shrinks from the fear that friends and strangers on the street will scorn her because her child is an idiot."[78]

During the 1950s, emerging research on the importance of the mother–infant bond began to question the wisdom of early institutionalization.[79] Several classic studies regarding institutionalized children described the deleterious effects of maternal deprivation on child development.[80] These studies portrayed the mother as critical to optimal early development and led a number of researchers to revisit the wisdom of infant institutionalization. Over the course of the late 1950s and 1960s, physicians increasingly recommended that children remain at home with their mothers at least for the first few years of life prior to being placed in a residential facility.[81] In cases where the mother was too emotionally fragile to fulfill her maternal duty, foster homes and small boarding houses were considered viable—although suboptimal—alternatives for care of affected children. Despite these recommendations, infant institutionalization remained extremely common.

While doctors urged early placement, most institutions were not designed for babies or the specialized care that they required. Families frantically trying to find a place for their infants felt frustrated by the severe shortage of facilities willing to care for infants and young children. Some institutions responded by adding nurseries but were unable to keep up with the demand. Many reported severe crib shortages. Relative affordability of public institutions contrasted sharply with expense of private facilities. Unable to secure a spot for a newborn in a public institution, some parents resorted to placing their babies in privately run nurseries or boarding homes—a very expensive option beyond what many could afford. In addition, privately run businesses were unregulated, so quality varied considerably. For most families, the public institution was the only tenable option, and parents had no choice but to place their child on a waiting list and hope a space would come available.

Institutional records suggest that issues of class, race, education, and ethnicity all influenced the decision to institutionalize. Physicians working at the Pacific State Hospital wrote that "professional people, and those with moderate to large incomes, usually make the choice of placement in spite of recommendations to the contrary. Families with less means and different value judgments about intellectual inadequacy will keep the child at home. The Oriental, Mexican-American, and Negro families rarely place at birth."[82] For reasons that may have been both cultural and financial, immigrant and African American children were disproportionately underrepresented. Dr. Sidney Werkman reported that while foreign-born parents kept their children with Down syndrome at home 80 percent of the time, native-born parents did so only about 40 percent of the time.[83] Dr. Kenneth Downey noted that more educated parents tended to institutionalize younger children and infants.[84] These families, he surmised, "have great hopes and aspirations for their children stressing not only socialization as an internalization of norms but also socialization as preparation for entering the higher levels of formal education. The diagnosis of retardation quickly shatters these hopes and aspirations."[85] Institutionalized children with Down syndrome disproportionately hailed from white, middle-class families, but it is hard to determine the degree to which these demographic trends reflected doctors' advice, parental preference, societal pressure, institutional rules, or some combination of these factors. The recognition that white, educated, wealthier parents tended to choose institutionalization additionally reflected the gender norms embedded in midcentury values of the upwardly mobile father and the mother intent on raising a crew of bright children.

The impulse to institutionalize seemed oblivious to mounting evidence about crowded conditions, high mortality rates, and abysmal developmental outcomes of institutionalized children.[86] Reports of squalid, congested conditions in state institutions began to emerge in the 1940s.[87] Journalist Edith Stern visited several state institutions and called them "little more than wretched zoos."[88] Potent sources of infection and neglect, these facilities were inhospitable environments for particularly vulnerable infants. The first year of residence was especially risky, with newly admitted children experiencing astronomical mortality rates ranging from 11 to 50 percent.[89] George Tarjan, the superintendent of the Pacific State Hospital in Pomona, California, complained that doctors did not caution parents about the "difficult adjustment period" after admission or about risk of death in the first year for patients with Down syndrome.[90] And despite research from the 1940s that showed "normal" children who had been institutionalized since birth withered developmentally, few pediatricians questioned the wisdom of subjecting infants with Down syndrome to a similar fate.[91]

As a result, throughout the 1950s, most physicians seemed unaware of or unmoved by the challenges of poor childhood survival in an institution. Physicians working in institutions published articles exploring the unhealthy conditions and strikingly poor health outcomes in these facilities, but their message was barely alluded to in the mainstream pediatric literature for most of the 1950s and 1960s. Some of the doctors working at these facilities tried to sound the alarm and urge fellow doctors to delay recommending institutionalization. But parents worried that it would be harder to give up their child after they had taken him or her home. And this was often framed as particularly difficult for mothers, although surveys of parents showed that fathers often struggled as well.[92]

Even as doctors continued to press for institutionalization, some parents began to question the wisdom of this path. Starting back in the 1930s, some parents had found each other and formed support groups.[93] By 1950, many of these collectives coalesced to form the National Association for Retarded Children (NARC), now known as The ARC.[94] During their meetings, parents shared stories about raising children at home, making the difficult decision to institutionalize, and learning their child's diagnosis. Some recalled positive conversations with compassionate physicians, but many voiced resentment about their experience. Parents recalled the diagnosis conversation with startling accuracy, even when it had occurred many years earlier. One researcher claimed that meetings with doctors were so emotionally charged they became indelible in parents' memories and that their recall was over 80 percent accurate.[95] Parents complained bitterly about the negative language their doctors used—particularly words like idiot, moron, imbecile, and mongol that had once had specific scientific meanings but had now slipped into a disparaging vernacular. Parents coping with Down syndrome urged the medical profession to adopt more neutral terms.[96] They recalled callous, hurried conversations, sometimes held over the phone, and the feeling of being dismissed.[97] Some told shocking stories of their children being called a monster or no better than a pet.[98] Parents also conveyed the horror of discovering the diagnosis weeks, months, and even years later, often because someone had slipped up and assumed they realized their child was "a mongol." They resented not being told the diagnosis as a couple and not being allowed to hold their baby, as well as being told the litany of ways that a child with Down syndrome would threaten their marriage, family, and social standing.

As these parents spoke with each other, and as they heard from parents who refused to institutionalize, they began to recognize that Down syndrome was not as horrible as had been billed. Parents who cared for their child at home described a fully loved and integrated family member who had defied the doctors' predictions and learned to walk, talk, and develop. Their children had refuted the doctor's dire warnings that the child would harm their family. Another striking feature involved the voices emerging from these parent groups—voices emanating from both men and women who frequently saw their experience as a shared one. These couples asked to be told the diagnosis together, rather than separately. They wanted to be seen as partners who were raising a family together. Inspired to help new parents, support groups cooperated with researchers in studies examining their experiences and recommending improvement—the first of which appeared in 1954.[99]

In the 1950s, even some professional advice encouraged the mother and father to act—and be treated—as partners in deciding the future of their child. Benjamin Spock's advice in the 1946 first edition of his classic, *The Common Sense Book of Baby and Child Care*, typified professional consensus at the time. "If the family can afford to place the Mongolian baby in a special home, it is usually recommended that this be done right after birth," he wrote. "Then the parents will not become too wrapped up in a child who will never develop very far."[100] But by 1957, Spock's message suggested that institutionalization was the parents' decision, saying, "Some doctors recommend to parents who can afford it that the baby be cared for in a private nursing home from birth, so that they will not become over attached to a child who is not likely to develop far. . . . This may be the better plan in some families, not in others. I think parents should take their time in coming to a decision."[101] The importance of Spock's subtle shift cannot be underestimated. His book was considered a "bible" by most mothers of that generation, and his word was the law.

In the early 1950s, as parent groups became more vocal, a story about mongolism became a bestseller when Dale Evans Rogers published a memoir about raising her daughter with Down syndrome.[102] Known as the "Queen of the West" and the "King of the Cowboys," Dale Evans and her husband Roy Rogers were megastars of movies, radio, and TV who had met on the set and married in 1947. Their daughter, Robin, was born in 1950.[103] Dale recalled that in the days after her birth, she was allowed to see Robin less frequently than other mothers on the maternity ward. In addition, the nurses seemed avoidant. Finally, one nurse urged her, "Tell your doctor to tell you the truth." The doctors had first informed their business manager and later Roy that Robin had Down syndrome and that they recommended immediate institutionalization. The physicians expressed the typical concerns about raising Robin at home—that Dale would be over-whelmed with Robin's care and would neglect their other children. After con-sulting a number of physicians, only one of whom advised them to take Robin home, Dale and Roy decided not to follow the doctors' advice. They hired full-time nurses to care for Robin and built a separate home on their ranch for that purpose. Concerned about the stigma associated with Down syndrome, Robin's diagnosis remained secret from everyone but their closest friends.

Two days before her second birthday, Robin died. Grief-ridden, Dale found inspiration in *The Child Who Never Grew*, the autobiographical depiction of Pearl Buck's search for help for her daughter, later found to have phenylketon-uria.[104] Buck ultimately chose institutionalization. Dale felt that Robin's story was more affirming and needed to be told. Deeply religious, Dale believed that Robin had been a heavenly messenger bringing their family closer to God and to each other. She also believed that their story of raising a disabled child at home would appeal to other parents in a similar situation, and so she decided to tell it.

A small religious press published Dale's book, *Angel Unaware*, in 1954. Thousands of parents wrote her expressing their gratitude for the way she put words to their family's difficult experience. Readers thanked her for expressing the truth about raising a developmentally disabled child. *Angel Unaware* was on the bestseller list for months and launched Dale's career as an inspirational religious writer.[105] Notably, *Angel Unaware* was the first book written by a par-ent about raising a child with Down syndrome. Dale and Roy preached Robin's story throughout their careers at religious gatherings and believed they had inspired many parents to opt against institutionalization and others to stop hid-ing their children. The book's royalties supported parent groups, including NARC, as well as medical research.

Robin Rogers's story is analogous to those of Neil Erikson and Daniel Miller, given the fact that the fathers were informed first, the assumptions that an infant with Down syndrome would be deleterious to marriage and siblings, and the clear message from physicians that institutionalization was preferable to home care. But the Rogers' choice to reject the path outlined by their doctors, and Dale's decision to publicize their experience, represented a cultural and perceptual shift that was beginning to gain momentum. Roy and Dale resisted efforts to embody roles their doctors expected of them. The couple made a decision to raise Robin together and trusted that their other children would be able to adapt to a fragile sibling with Down syndrome. Their story appealed to members of parent groups who, like the Rogers, felt that viable alternatives to institutionalization existed.

Angel Unaware was a popular representation of a much broader movement calling for new ways to envision Down syndrome and other forms of intellectual delay. Like the research emerging from parent groups, *Angel Unaware* offered an alternative perspective that challenged traditional expectations for mothers and fathers. Although the book drew on a conservative, Christian interpretation of the ultimate meaning of intellectual delay in a world that appeared to reject people with intellectual delay, the story also espoused a radical idea—that parents and families could endure this type of unexpected hardship together and benefit substantially from the experience. While both were rocked by the reality that Robin was not the perfect baby they had expected, and while both grieved that loss, they believed in their ability to raise their daughter. Dale and Roy epitomized conservative Christianity and reinforced traditional gender roles in private and on screen, but they also believed in facing challenges together. Dale was, after all, a career woman juggling the demands of being a mother, wife, and a holding down a demanding and very public job. Both on and off the screen, she and Roy were partners.

The increased awareness of parents' experiences of raising a child with Down syndrome prompted physician recommendations and standard care to evolve. Beginning in the mid-1950s, several organizations, including the American Association on Mental Deficiency, the Expert Committee on the Mentally Subnormal Child of the World Health Organization,[106] and the Group for the Advancement of Psychiatry, endorsed more hopeful, parent-centered approaches to relaying the diagnosis of Down syndrome. Doctors urged each other to adopt milder language, to be more hopeful, and to see the child as an accepted and integral family member, rather than as a failure or threat.[107] Research published in the 1960s found that most siblings fared well and marriages did not inevitably end in divorce.[108] Studies comparing children raised at home and those in institutions showed markedly improved developmental outcomes among home-reared individuals and provided developmental rationale for postponing institutionalization for a number of years at least.[109] Change did not happen overnight; some physicians remained firmly entrenched in the early institutionalization camp and, along with many parents, expressed their concerns in opinionated, gendered language. But the tide was starting to turn. Exemplifying this shift was Joseph Weingold, the executive director of the Association for the Help of Retarded Children and a father of a child with Down syndrome. Addressing a symposium composed of prominent physicians and researchers, he told his family's story of their son Jonny—"an altogether delightful little boy." He felt that children with Down syndrome were starting to get the attention they needed. "The answer to mongolism is right outside the door," he continued, "We are here forging the key to open the door—through understanding and the recognition of the worth of a mongoloid child as an individual, and his dignity as a human being."[110]

Acknowledgment

The author would like to acknowledge anonymous reviewers and especially Sarah T. Rice, MD, who provided key research and analysis for this project.

Notes

1. Barbara Eisold, *In the Shadow of Fame: A Memoir by the Daughter of Erik Erikson* (book review), *Psychoanalysis*, Spring 2005, 37–40, http://www.apadivisons.org/division-39/publications/reviews/shadow-fame.aspx (accessed April 25, 2018). Sue Erikson Bloland, *In the Shadow of Fame: A Memoir by the Daughter of Erik H. Erikson* (New York: Viking, 2005), 20–27.

2. Mark Edmundson, "Psychoanalysis, American Style," book review of Lawrence J. Friedman, *Identity's Architect: A Biography of Erik H. Erikson* (New York: Scribner, 1999), *New York Times*, August 22, 1999, https://archive.nytimes.com/www.nytimes.com/books/99/08/22/reviews/990822.22edmundt.html?scp=7&sq=theodor%2520w%2520adorno&st=cse (accessed April 25, 2018).

3. Suzanna Andrews, "Arthur Miller's Missing Act," *Vanity Fair* http://www.vanityfair.com/culture/2007/09/miller200709 (accessed December 12, 2017).

4. Maureen Dowd, "What's Zeus, Really? He's Just a Father," *New York Times*, March 15, 2018.

5. Maureen Downd, "What's Zeus, Really? He's Just a Father," *New York Times*, March 15, 2018.

6. Alfred White Franklin, "The Care of the Mongol Baby: The First Phase," *The Lancet* 271 (1958): 256–58, p. 256.

7. A. H. Parmelee, "Management of Mongolism in Childhood," *International Record of Medicine and General Practice Clinics* 169 (June 1956): 358–61, p. 359.

8. The crisis motif was very common. See, for example, James G. Hughes, *Synopsis of Pediatrics*, 2nd ed. (St. Louis, MO: CV Mosby, 1967), 70, and Bernard Farber, "Perceptions of Crisis and Related Variables in the Impact of a Retarded Child on the Mother," *Journal of Health and Human Behavior* 1 (1960): 108–18.

9. John Langdon Down, "Observations on an Ethnic Classification of Idiots," *London Hospital Reports* 3 (1866): 259–62.

10. David Wright, *Downs: The History of a Disability* (Oxford: Oxford University Press, 2011), 48.

11. Down, "Observations on an Ethnic Classification of Idiots."

12. Wright's book addresses the importance and meaning of the various names that have been used for Down syndrome. See especially Wright, *Downs*, 115–45, chap. 4.

13. Throughout his career, Clemens Benda, a leading authority on Down syndrome, tried to make a case an endocrinological etiology for the syndrome. See, for example, Clemens E. Benda, *The Child with Mongolism (Congenital Acromicria)* (New York: Grune and Stratton, 1960).

14. Wright, *Downs*, 10; Jerome Lejeune, Marthe Gautier, and M. Raymond Turpin, "Etude des chromosomes somatiques de neuf enfants mongoliens," *Academie des Sciences* 248 (1959): 1721–22.

15. Wright, *Downs*, 115–19.

16. Martin S. Pernick, *The Black Stork: Eugenics and the Death of "Defective" Babies in American Medicine and Motion Pictures since 1915* (Oxford: Oxford University Press, 1996).

17. Leila Zenderland, "The Parable of the Kallikak Family: Explaining the Meaning of Heredity in 1912," in *Mental Retardation in America: A Historical Reader*, ed. Steven Noll and James Trent Jr. (New York: New York University Press, 2003), 165–85.

18. J. C. and Helen Furnas, "Ill-Finished Children," *Saturday Evening Post* 218 (1945): 17+, quotation on 17.

19. Sidney A. Halpern, *American Pediatrics: The Social Dynamics of Professionalism, 1880–1980* (Berkeley: University of California Press, 1988).

20. Rima D. Apple, *Perfect Motherhood* (New Brunswick, NJ: Rutgers University Press, 2006); Rima Apple, "Constructing Mothers: Scientific Motherhood in the Nineteenth and Twentieth Centuries," in *Mothers and Medicine: Readings in American History*, ed. Rima D. Apple and Janet Golden (Columbus: Ohio State University Press, 1997), 90–110.

21. During the 1940s, life expectancy at birth rose four years. U.S. Department of Health, Education and Welfare, Children's Bureau, *Health Services for Mentally Retarded Children: A Progress Report, 1956–60* (Washington, D.C.: U.S. Government Printing Office, 1961), 1.

22. Lynn Z. Bloom, *Doctor Spock: Biography of a Conservative Radical* (Indianapolis, IN: Bobbs-Merrill, 1972), 116. For more on the impact of Spock's child care manual, see Nancy Pottisham Weiss, "Mother, the Invention of Necessity: Dr. Benjamin Spock's Baby and Child Care," in *Growing Up in America: Children in Historical Perspective*, ed. N. Ray Hiner and Joseph M. Hawes (Urbana: University of Illinois Press, 1985), 283–303, and Janet Golden, *Babies Made Us Modern: How Infants Brought America into the Twentieth Century* (Cambridge: Cambridge University Press, 2018).

23. Bloom, *Doctor Spock*, 116.

24. Jeffrey P. Brosco, Michael I. Seider, and Angela C. Dunn, "Universal Newborn Screening and Adverse Medical Outcomes: A Historical Note," *Mental Retardation and Developmental Disabilities Research Reviews* 12 (2006): 262–69, p. 265.

25. Leslie J. Reagan, *Dangerous Pregnancies: Mothers, Disabilities, and Abortion in Modern America* (Berkeley: University of California Press, 2010).

26. Reagan, 182–86.

27. Diane B. Paul and Jeffrey P. Brosco, *The PKU Paradox: A Short History of a Genetic Disease* (Baltimore: Johns Hopkins University Press, 2013).

28. Many articles expressed the theme of hopelessness in the diagnosis of mental retardation in general and Down syndrome in particular. For an early example, see Arnold Gesell, "Developmental Diagnosis in Infancy," *New England Journal of Medicine* 192

(1925): 1058–60, and, almost sixty years later, Simon Olshansky, Gertrude C. Johnson, and Leon Sternfeld, "Attitudes of Some GP's toward Institutionalizing Mentally Retarded Children," *Mental Retardation* 1 (1963): 18–20, 57–59, p. 19.

29. Experts warned about grasping for straws with unfounded therapies for many forms of childhood mental delay. See George Tarjan, "The Role of the Primary Physician in Mental Retardation," *California Medicine* 102 (1965): 423; Hyman Goldstein, "Treatment of Mongolism and Non-Mongoloid Mental Retardation in Children," *Archives of Pediatrics* 71 (1954): 77.

30. Elaine Tyler May, *Homeward Bound: American Families in the Cold War Era* (New York: Basic Books, 1988); Reagan, *Dangerous Pregnancies.*

31. Janice Brockley, "Rearing the Child Who Never Grew: Ideologies of Parenting and Intellectual Disability in American History," in *Mental Retardation in America: A Historical Reader*, ed. Steven Noll and James W. Trent Jr. (New York: New York University Press, 2004), 130–64.

32. On Spock, see Golden, *Babies Made Us Modern* and Michael Zuckerman, "Dr. Spock: The Confidence Man," in *The Family in History*, ed. Charles E. Rosenberg (Philadelphia: University of Pennsylvania Press, 1975), 179–207.

33. Jeffrey P. Baker, "Autism in 1959: Joey the Mechanical Boy," *Pediatrics* 125 (2010): 1101–3.

34. Fanny Stang, "Parent Guidance and the Mentally Retarded Child," *Public Health* 71 (1957–58): 234–36, p. 235.

35. Goldstein, "Treatment of Mongolism and Non-Mongoloid Mental Retardation," 95.

36. Comment by Dr. Edward Shaw in F. H. Stewart, S. Clifford, L. Hill, and H. Bakwin, "Early Home Care or Institution for the Retarded Child," *Journal of Pediatrics* 42 (1953): 396–400, p. 397. Brennemann's actual position is more difficult to determine. In his 1943 "Approach to the Parents on a Subnormal Child," he stated, "Few mothers will consent to sending away a baby, and few institutions will accept one at that age, but the thought has been planted and it will grow as occasion warrants. I know of only one baby, a Mongolian idiot in a well-to-do home, who, after confirmation of the diagnosis by several pediatricians, was transferred to a foster home shortly after birth." Joseph Brennemann Papers, Division of Library and Archival Services, American Academy of Pediatrics, Elk Grove Village, IL.

37. C. Anderson Aldrich and Mary M. Aldrich, *Babies are Human Beings: An Interpretation of Growth* (New York: Macmillan, 1938). For more on Aldrich and his popular child care manual, see Golden, *Babies Made Us Modern*, 181–82.

38. C. Anderson Aldrich, "Preventive Medicine and Mongolism," *American Journal of Mental Deficiency* 52 (October 1947): 127–29, p. 128. Many other writers agreed with Aldrich. See, for instance, Franklin, "The Care of the Mongol Baby," 257.

39. Aldrich, "Preventive Medicine and Mongolism," 128.

40. Aldrich, 128.

41. Aldrich, 127–29.

42. Doctors appeared to gravitate toward fathers in other areas as well. See Kathleen E. Bachynski, "'The Duty of Their Elders'—Doctors, Coaches, and the Framing of Youth Football's Health Risks, 1950s–1960s," *Journal of the History of Medicine and Allied Sciences* 74 (2019): 167–91.

43. Richard B. Tudor, "What to Tell Parents of a Retarded Child," *The Lancet* 79 (1959): 196–98, p. 198. Siegried A. Centerwall and Willard R. Centerwall, "A Study of Children with Mongolism Reared in the Home Compared to Those Reared Away from the Home," *Pediatrics* 25 (1960): 678–85, p. 679.

44. Charles Ludwig and Marshall Porter, "The Physician, the Parent and the Retarded Child," discussion by Arthur Parmelee, *California Medicine* 80 (1954): 394–97, p. 396.

45. Sidney Werkman, John A. Washington, and J. William Oberman, "Symposium: The Physician and Mongolism," *Clinical Proceedings—Children's Hospital of the District of Columbia* 17 (1961): 42–49, p. 47.

46. Centerwall and Centerwall stated that "in 100 percent of the cases the reason which the parents gave for desiring placement in the neonatal period was that the doctor advised it." Centerwall and Centerwall, "A Study of Children," 683.

47. Werkman et al., "Symposium," 43.

48. Olshansky et al., "Attitudes of Some GP's," 19.

49. Kenneth J. Downey, "Parents' Reasons for Institutionalizing Severely Mentally Retarded Children," *Journal of Health and Human Behavior* 6, no. 3 (Autumn 1965): 147–55, p. 150.

50. Clifford G. Grulee and R. Cannon Eley, *The Child in Health and Disease: A Textbook for Students and Practitioners of Medicine* (Baltimore: Williams and Wilkins Co., 1948), 724. See also, Olshansky et al., "Attitudes of Some GP's," 19.

51. Malcolm J. Farrell, "The Adverse Effects of Early Institutionalization of Mentally Subnormal Children," *AMA Journal of Diseases of Children* 91 (1956): 278–81, p. 278.

52. Farrell, 278. It was also common for doctors to suggest that the parents tell their family and friends that the baby had died. Martha Eliot, MD, chief of the Children's Bureau, recalled seeing a toddler in an institution whose parents made that decision, only to discover later that "the child was not a monster." Farrell, 278–79.

53. Centerwall and Centerwall, "A Study of Children," 683. A fictionalized story along these lines is Kim Edwards, *The Memory Keeper's Daughter* (New York: Viking, 2005).

54. Donald H. Jolly, "When Should the Seriously Retarded Infant be Institutionalized?" *American Journal of Mental Retardation* 57 (1953): 632–36.

55. Judith Walzer Leavitt, *Make Room for Daddy: The Journey from Waiting Room to Birthing Room* (Chapel Hill: University of North Carolina Press, 2009).

56. Leo Kanner, "Parents' Feelings about Retarded Children," *American Journal of Mental Deficiency* 57 (1953): 375–83, p. 382.

57. Janet Carr, "Mongolism: Telling the Parents," *Developmental Medicine & Child Neurology* 12 (1970): 213–21, p. 219. In a letter to the editor, K. A. Evans wrote about parents' recall of being told their child's diagnosis, saying, "I am struck by the extremely vivid and sometimes quite horrifying memories they have of being 'told'. Many of them can relive in detail this traumatic experience even after 10 and 15 years." K. A. Evans, "Mentally Handicapped Children," letter to the editor, *The Lancet* 279 (1962): 974.

58. Valerie Cowie, "Genetic Counselling," in "Symposium: The Handicapped Child [Abridged]" *Proceedings of the Royal Society of Medicine* 59 (1966): 149–50, p. 150.

59. In the study, one physician's actions were not included. Wellington Hung and Nicholas P. Haritos, "The Mongoloid Newborn: Problems Faced by the Pediatrician and Family," *Clinical Proceedings, Children's Hospital, Washington, DC* 17 (1961): 31–42, pp. 32 and 34.

60. Franklin, "The Care of the Mongol Baby," 258.

61. T. A. Fortune, letter to the editor, "Mentally Handicapped Children: The Parents' View," *The Lancet* 279 (March 3, 1962): 482–83, p. 482.

62. Ridgely Hunt, "The Unfinished Children," *Chicago Tribune*, February 12, 1967, http://archives.chicagotribune.com/1967/02/12/page/209/article/the-unfinished-children (accessed June 28, 2017).

63. William F. Gayton and Linda Walker, "Down Syndrome: Informing the Parents, a Study of Parental Preferences," *American Journal of Diseases of Children* 127 (1974): 510–12, p. 512.

64. Stanley W. Wright and George Tarjan, "Mental Retardation: A Review for Pediatricians," *American Journal of Diseases of Children* 105 (1963): 511–26, p. 522.

65. Wright and Tarjan, 522.

66. Wright and Tarjan, 522.

67. Armand Matheny Antomarria, "'Who Should Survive? One of the Choices on Our Conscience': Mental Retardation and the History of Contemporary Bioethics," *Kennedy Institute of Ethics Journal* 16 (2006): 205–24.

68. *Who Should Survive*, a 1971 film sponsored by the Joseph P. Kennedy Jr. Foundation, reenacted the case of a newborn with Down syndrome and duodenal atresia who was allowed to starve to death in the hospital nursery when his parents declined corrective surgery. https://mn.gov/mnddc/ada-legacy/who-should-survive.html; Antommaria, "Who Should Survive?"

69. Ludwig and Porter, "The Physician, the Parent and the Retarded Child," 397.

70. Alastair Beddie and Humphry Osmond, "Mothers, Mongols, and Mores," *Canadian Medical Journal* 73 (1955): 167–70.

71. Jolly, "When Should the Seriously Retarded Infant Be Institutionalized?" 632, 633. He attributed this trend to earlier diagnosis, the convincing advice of consultants (i.e., pediatricians), and intense community pressure to institutionalize.

72. Jolly, 634.

73. Jolly, 635.

74. Jolly, 633.

75. Centerwall and Centerwall, "A Study of Children," 679.

76. Tudor, "What to Tell Parents of a Retarded Child," 198.

77. Elizabeth R. Kramm, *Families of Mongoloid Children* (Washington, D.C.: Department of Health, Education, and Welfare, Children's Bureau, 1963), 30.

78. Ridgely Hunt, "The Unfinished Children," *Chicago Tribune*, February 12, 1967, http://archives.chicagotribune.com/1967/01/12/page/209/article/the-unfinished -children.

79. See Wellington Hung and Nicholas P. Haritos, "The Mongoloid Newborn: Problems Faced by the Pediatrician and Family," *Clinical Proceedings, Children's Hospital, Washington, DC* 17 (1961): 31–42, p. 38.

80. R. A. Spitz, "Hospitalism: Inquiry into Genesis of Psychiatric Conditions in Early Childhood," *Psychoanalytic Study of the Child*, 1 (1945): 53–74; Farrell, "Adverse Effects of Early Institutionalization"; J. Bowlby, "Maternal Care and Mental Health," *WHO Monograph*, series no. 2 (Geneva: Palais des Nations, 1951).

81. Robert B. Kugel and David Reque, "A Comparison of Mongoloid Children," *JAMA* 175 (1961): 959–61, p. 961.

82. Wright and Tarjan, "Mental Retardation," 523.

83. Werkman et al., "Symposium," 48. He reported that mixed foreign- and native-born parents kept their Down syndrome children at home 60 percent of the time.

84. Kenneth J. Downey, "Parents' Reasons for Institutionalizing Severely Mentally Retarded Children," *Journal of Health and Human Behavior* 6 (Autumn 1965): 147–55, p. 149.

85. Kenneth J. Downey, "Parental Interest in the Institutionalized, Severely Mentally Retarded Child," *Social Problems* 11 (1963): 186–93, p. 192.

86. Brennemann felt that distance was good because it prevented frequent visits that could be painful for the parents. In 1954, California reported that it had 6,700 patients in state hospitals built for 5,600 and that an additional 3,000 were on the waiting list. Ludwig and Porter, "The Physician, the Parent and the Retarded Child," 394.

87. James W. Trent Jr., *Inventing the Feeble Mind: A History of Mental Retardation in the United States* (Berkeley: University of California Press, 1994).

88. Edith M. Stern, "Take Them Off the Human Scrap Heap," *Woman's Home Companion* 75 (August 1948): 32–33+, p. 32.

89. Richard A. Kurtz, "Sex and Age Trends in Admissions to an Institution for the Mentally Retarded, 1910–1959," *Nebraska State Medical Journal* 52 (1967): 134–43. This institution reported that 34 percent of all patients under five admitted 1955–1959 died. At Pacific State Hospital in Pomona, California, between 1948 and 1952, close to 20 percent of the patients with "mongolism" died in the first six months and close to 40 percent had died by the time they had been in the hospital four years. These were predominantly ages zero to four at the time of admission. See George Tarjan, Stanley W. Wright, Morton Kramer, Philip H. Person, and Richard Morgan, "The Natural History of Mental Deficiency in a State Hospital," *A.M.A. Journal of Diseases of Children* 96 (July 1958): 64–70, p. 67. Richard A. Kurtz and Wolf Wolfensberger, "Separation Experiences of Residents in an Institution for the Mentally Retarded: 1910–1959," *American Journal of Mental Deficiency* 74 (1969): 389–96, reported that infants admitted between 1950 and 1959 had a 51 percent mortality rate and claimed that at other institutions, the mortality rates were similarly high.

90. Tarjan et al., "The Natural History of Mental Deficiency in a State Hospital," 68–69.

91. Lauretta Bender, "Infants Reared in Institutions," *Bulletin of the Child Welfare League of America* 24 (September 1945): 1–4.

92. Downey, "Parents' Reasons for Institutionalizing Severely Mentally Retarded Children."

93. Kathleen W. Jones, "Education for Children with Mental Retardation: Parent Activism, Public Policy, and Family Ideology in the 1950s," in *Mental Retardation in America: A Historical Reader*, ed. Steven Noll and James W. Trent Jr. (New York: NYU Press, 2004), 322–50; Katherine Castles, "'Nice, Average Americans': Postwar Parents' Groups and the Defense of the Normal Family," in *Mental Retardation in America: A Historical Reader*, ed. Steven Noll and James W. Trent Jr. (New York: NYU Press, 2004), 351–70.

94. On the various names that the organization has used, see www.thearc.org/who-we -are/history-name-change.

95. Janet Carr, "Six Weeks to Twenty-One Years Old: A Longitudinal Study of Children with Down's Syndrome and Their Families," Third Jack Tizard Memorial Lecture, *Journal of Child Psychology and Psychiatry* 29 (1988): 407–31.

96. In 1959, Dr. Jack Edelstein described the system of scientific nomenclature that had been in place for over half a century: morons had IQs of 50–70, imbeciles of 20–50, and idiots of <20. J. P. Edelstein and S. H. Frazier, "Current Practices in General Medicine: 4. Parental Counseling in Mental Retardation," *Proceedings of the Staff Meetings of the Mayo Clinic* 34 (May 13, 1959): 247–55. See also Charlotte H. Waskowitz, "The Parents of Retarded Children Speak for Themselves," *Journal of Pediatrics* 54 (1959): 319–29, p. 324.

97. Richard Koch, Betty V. Graliker, Russell Sands, and Arthur H. Parmelee, "Attitude Study of Parents with Mentally Retarded Children: I. Evaluation of Parental

Satisfaction with the Medical Care of a Retarded Child," *Pediatrics* 23 (1959): 582–84, p. 583, and Waskowitz, "The Parents of Retarded Children Speak for Themselves," 320–23.

98. Israel Zwerling, "Initial Counseling of Parents with Mentally Retarded Children," *Journal of Pediatrics* 44, no. 4 (April 1954): 469–79, p. 471.

99. Zwerling, "Initial Counseling of Parents"; H. B., Editor's Column, "Parents of the Mentally Retarded Child," *Journal of Pediatrics*, 44, no. 4 (April 1954): 486–87. For other studies of parents' reactions to the diagnosis, see Martha Taylor Schipper, "The Child with Mongolism in the Home," *Pediatrics* 24 (1959): 134–44 and Waskowitz, "The Parents of Retarded Children Speak for Themselves." Waskowitz noted that only 25 percent of the parents felt their interaction with physicians was satisfactory (p. 322).

100. Benjamin Spock, *The Common Sense Book of Baby and Child Care* (New York: Duell, Sloan and Pearce, 1946), 502–3, quoted in Rima D. Apple, *Perfect Motherhood* (New Brunswick, NJ: Rutgers University Press, 2006), 131.

101. Benjamin Spock, *Dr. Benjamin Spock's Baby and Child Care*, quoted in Apple, *Perfect Motherhood*, 593.

102. H. Hughes Evans and Sarah T. Rice, "Angel Unaware and Down Syndrome Awareness," *Pediatrics* 142 (2018): e20173553.

103. The story of her diagnosis has been told in numerous books written by and about the Rogers, and the story varies a bit. Dale Evans Rogers, *Angel Unaware* (Grand Rapids, MI: Revell, 1953); Elise Miller Davis, *The Answer Is God: The Inspiring Story of Dale Evans and Roy Rogers* (New York: McGraw-Hill, 1955); Maxine Garrison, *The Angel Spreads Her Wings* (Westwood, CT: Fleming H. Revell Co., 1956); Roy Rogers and Dale Evans, *Happy Trails: Our Life Story* (New York: Simon & Schuster, 1994).

104. Pearl S. Buck, *The Child Who Never Grew*, 2nd ed. (Bethesda, MD: Woodbine House, 1992 [New York: John Day, 1950]). See also Paul and Brosco, *The Paradox of PKU*.

105. Rogers and Evans, *Happy Trails*; Dale Evans Rogers, *In the Hands of the Potter* (Nashville, TN: Thomas Nelson, 1994), among others.

106. Farrell, "Adverse Effects of Early Institutionalization," 278–79.

107. The first report of parent reactions was Zwerling, "Initial Counseling of Parents with Mentally Retarded Children," which was accompanied by an editorial: H.B. "Parents of the Mentally Retarded Child." See also Schipper, "The Child with Mongolism in the Home," 141–43, and Gerald Solomons, "What Do You Tell the Parents of a Retarded Child?" *Clinical Pediatrics* 4 (1965): 227–32.

108. B. Farber, "Effects of a Severely Mentally Retarded Child on Family Integration," *Monographs of the Society for Research in Child Development*, serial no. 71, 24 (1959): 1–112.

109. Centerwall and Centerwall, "A Study of Children," 685.

110. Joseph T. Weingold, "Rehabilitation of the Mongoloid Child: Introductory Remarks," in Mongolism: A Symposium, *Quarterly Review of Pediatrics* (May, August, November 1953 issues), in Clemens Benda papers, Box 6, Folder 234, Center for the History of Medicine, Francis A. Countway Library of Medicine.

Chapter 4

Making Children into Boys and Girls

Gender Role in 1950s Pediatric Endocrinology

Sandra Eder

Gender was and is not only an organizing principle in American pediatrics, as this volume argues. The current sex/gender binary was actually first formulated in the 1950s within the new subspecialty of pediatric endocrinology.[1] A team of pediatricians, psychologists, psychiatrists, and surgeons developed a new concept of sex that separated children's biological sex from the social sex in which they were raised and from a gender role they learned and consequently inhabited. They did so with the intention to help medical practitioners assess and decide on the sex of children with disorders of sexual development (DSD) or intersex who they encountered in their clinical practice. Their recommendations still affect the lives of these children to this day.

Humans come in all variations, of course, and some children are born with or develop a variation from what we commonly understand as male and female. Often their sexual anatomy is only slightly different from what we perceive as standard male or female bodies, but sometimes their unusual anatomies result in confusion and debates about whether they should be considered male or female.[2] These individuals have been referred to as hermaphrodites in the past. Today, "intersex" and "DSD" are broader terms to describe children born with sex-atypical gonads, hormones, chromosomes, or genitals.[3] The Johns Hopkins Hospital was a research and treatment hub for such patients, and most cases were seen by urologist Hugh Hampton Young, director of the Brady Urological Institute at the Johns Hopkins Hospital until his retirement in 1942.[4] By then, more and more of these patients were referred to the Pediatric Endocrinology Clinic at the Harriet Lane Home for Invalid Children, which was situated on the Johns Hopkins Hospital grounds.

The concern with determining a person's true sex was not a new one. Since the late nineteenth century, sex had become increasingly medicalized, and many physicians shared an interest in studying and classifying cases of hermaphroditism.[5] Relying on a classification system developed by German pathologist Theodor Albrecht Edwin Klebs in 1876, which divided hermaphrodites into true hermaphrodites and pseudohermaphrodites based upon their gonads, many American physicians postulated that they had the expertise to determine a person's "true" sex regardless of appearance, demeanor, or behavior. Whoever possessed testes was male and whoever had ovaries was female.[6] By the twentieth century, advances in anesthesia and surgery also made it easier for medical experts to determine a person's sex based on these categories and to perform surgery if they thought it necessary to align genitals to fit the gonadal sex.[7] At the same time, many physicians wondered what to do in cases where behavior and character did not follow the gonadal sex. Should these people remain in the sex they already lived in even if it was not their "true" (i.e., gonadal) sex?

Until the early twentieth century, these medical encounters were with adults or teenagers who often sought medical guidance for an unrelated ailment, such as a hernia or failure of menses to onset, and who were then consequently diagnosed as pseudohermaphrodites or intersex. By the 1950s, the concerns about sex determination had shifted from adult patients to infants and children. American childbirth had been thoroughly medicalized, and the majority of children in the United States were born in hospitals.[8] Accordingly, unusual genitalia or doubts about sex were registered at a much earlier age, and these infants and children were referred to specialists such as pediatric endocrinologists for diagnosis and treatment. A set of case studies from the 1940s had discussed cases in which children had—accidently—been raised in the "wrong sex" and as teenagers and young adults identified with the sex they had been raised in rather than their biological one.[9] Physicians increasingly recommended making decisions about a child's sex early and correctly in order to avoid future situations in which an adult's sex turned out to be "wrong" or doubtful. Convinced that children could only be either male or female, medical practitioners faced a twofold conundrum: how to actually determine sex correctly in infants (and thus to decide which of the now multiple sex categories such as gonads, hormonal sex, external genitalia, internal reproductive organs, and increasingly chromosomal sex[10] trumped the others) and whether to change the sex children already lived in if it did not match their biological sex. A team at the Pediatric Endocrinology Clinic of the Harriet Lane Home for Invalid Children on the Johns Hopkins Hospital Campus in Baltimore proposed an answer to this question, which replaced biological determination of sex with measurements of behavior and adjustment.

Redefining Sex

Pediatrician Lawson Wilkins established the first specialty clinic with a focus on pediatric endocrinology in 1935, before the subspecialty even existed as a clearly defined field and at a time when many respectable physicians still worried about the public frenzy and scientific controversies that had accompanied early endocrinology.[11] A second such clinic was established under Nathan Talbot at Massachusetts General Hospital in 1942. The evolution of pediatric endocrinology as a subspecialty was in part facilitated by the evolution of subspecialty-focused academic pediatric centers, the availability of funding for research through government and private sources, and the development of subspecialty-oriented national medical professional societies and journals promoting basic and clinical research.[12] By the early 1950s, Wilkins's clinic in Baltimore was a hub of biomedical research and innovative clinical practice. He published the first textbook in the field, and many of the fellows he trained at his clinic established new pediatric endocrine training programs during the 1950s and 1960s in the United States.[13]

In the late 1930s, Wilkins developed an interest in congenital adrenal hyperplasia (CAH). Today we know that CAH occurs when the genetic "recipe" for making cortisol in the adrenal glands is not working. This causes synthesis and excretion of an androgen precursor, leading to virilization in utero and continuing after birth. In severe cases, the adrenals do not produce the hormone aldosterone, which leads to salt and water loss, and in these cases, the conditions may be life-threatening. Children are often sexually precocious and grow at an accelerated rate. Wilkins's first case of CAH in 1938 was not a girl with symptoms of pseudohermaphroditism but a little boy who passed away shortly after he was admitted to the Harriet Lane Home Clinic. Thus, one of his main concerns for both male and female patients was to prevent life-threatening symptoms such as salt loss.[14] He was, however, also concerned with the (very much) not life-threatening ones. In girls and women, CAH was considered a condition causing female pseudohermaphroditism and treated as such by clinicians and endocrinologists.[15] Girls with CAH often had male-appearing genitals and large clitorises, and they were sometimes thought to be boys at birth. If raised as girls, parents and pediatricians often expressed concern about the way their genitals looked and their increasingly masculine appearance.

In 1948, with no treatment insight for CAH, Wilkins discussed the question of sex with his colleagues at a conference on adrenal health at the annual meeting of the American Academy of Pediatrics.[16] Faced with the question of "how should we handle these patients who are female pseudohermaphrodites," he suggested to a fellow physician that it might be best for girls with CAH to be raised as boys and live as males.[17] Without available treatment, these girls would, he stressed, look increasingly male. Wilkins's suggestion seems curious given that he perceived these girls to be biological females, even though their genitals and appearance became male-appearing through the exposure to androgens in utero and after. Yet, their male appearance, he felt, would prevent them from fulfilling the social roles of women at the time. For example, Wilkins told his patients that they would never be able to marry or have children.[18] With that in mind, he thought that living as men would presumably give them some level of independence. A combination of testosterone during puberty, surgery to make their genitals look more convincingly male, and a hysterectomy and bilateral salpingo-oophorectomy (removal of both ovaries and fallopian tubes) would ensure a convincing male appearance. In the case of older girls with CAH who were already living as girls, he advised parents to keep raising them in the female sex and practitioners to adjust their bodies by amputating or shortening their clitorises.

In 1950, Wilkins started using cortisone as a therapeutic for children with CAH. Cortisone halted both the life-threatening aspects of the condition, including salt loss, as well as symptoms such as male-appearing genitals and increasing virilization in girls. By 1951, Wilkins was in the middle of a research program testing out various effects of the cortisone treatment for CAH patients.[19] For once he changed his recommendation to raise all female infants with CAH as girls. For this to work, it was crucial to diagnose CAH and consequently the sex of the child at birth. Genital surgery and long-term cortisone treatment would ensure their feminine appearance. But what about those girls who were already living as boys? Should they reverse the sex assignment of those girls who had so far been raised as boys, now that cortisone was available as treatment? To study this question and other related issues concerning sex assignment and psychological healthfulness, Wilkins hired a team consisting of psychiatrist Joan Hampson—a Johns Hopkins Medical School graduate who had just completed her residency in psychiatry at Henry Phipps Psychiatric Clinic—and John Money, a graduate student in clinical psychology at Harvard's Department of Social Relations, who was just writing up his dissertation, *Hermaphroditism: An Inquiry Into the Nature of a Human Paradox* (which he filed in 1952).[20]

Starting with Wilkins's CAH patients and expanding soon to patients with various diagnoses of "pseudohermaphroditism" at his clinic, Money and Hampson (later joined by her husband, fellow psychiatrist John Hampson) compared "assigned sex and sex of rearing" and five biological sex variables (external genital morphology, internal accessory reproductive structures, hormonal sex and secondary sexual characteristics, gonadal sex, and chromosomal sex) with a new term that Money claimed to have coined: "gender role." Gender was of course not a new term, but it had hitherto mostly been used as polite form of saying sex and in the grammatical sense. Social scientists at times, such as Margaret Mead and Talcott Parsons, referred to sex roles and psychiatrists discussed psychosexual development. Money's newly introduced term "gender role" described "all those things that a person says or does to disclose himself or herself as having the status of boy or man, girl or woman, respectively."[21] A child's orientation as male or female was established while growing up, they claimed. In a series of publications, the team concluded that gender role had no "innate, instinctive basis."[22] Rather, "the evidence of hermaphroditism" led them to conclude that children were sexually undifferentiated at birth and learned being masculine or feminine "in the course of the various experiences of growing up."[23]

Faced with contradictions between sex characteristics, anatomy, behavior, and self-perception, Wilkins's team offered a pragmatic solution for clinicians to the conundrum of finding a person's true sex: to choose the sex that promised the best outcome in terms of social adjustment and psychological healthiness. This was of course what Wilkins had already practiced when, before the introduction of cortisone, he recommended that female infants with CAH better be raised as males. Money and the Hampsons suggested that one could assign any of two sexes as early as possible, preferably the sex that would fit the external genitalia best. Afterward, parents should stick with this assignment firmly and act accordingly consistently around their child. A child's gender role was learned through experiences that were ineradicably imprinted on the child's mind in the first years of life, and therefore their sex should not be changed after age two-and-a-half. In order to make sex assignment convincing to parents and their children as well as their environment, they suggested using surgery to "reconstruct" the genitalia to fit the assigned sex of rearing, and thus the child's gender role, as early as possible. Infants could of course not consent to these invasive surgical procedures (their parents did), and many adult intersex activists have stressed the traumatic consequences these scarring and irreversible surgeries had. A great body of literature has revealed how the Hopkins recommendations, also known as "optimum gender of rearing" model of intersex case management, led to decades of treatment practices that normalized intersex patients into male and female bodies—with dire consequences for the patients' physical and emotional well-being.[24]

Assessing Gender

In terms of clinical practice, this was a treatment plan for the future, born out of a persistent clinical conviction that a person's true sex—male or female—had to be determined while pragmatically acknowledging the clinical experience of the previous decades that a person's true sex might not be the best sex for them. It seems ironic that biological determinism was replaced by a social determinism in which norms and roles served as assessment for a person's maleness and femaleness. How did pediatricians evaluate "gender role" and treatment success in these moments of sex assignment and after? How did they integrate the new idea of a learned gender role with the already existing notion of (mal)adjustment? In short, how was gender role assessed within clinical practice?

Wilkins and his team evaluated proper gender role through an assessment of femininity and masculinity that stemmed from clinical and parental observation of children's behavior and appearance. Most notably, sex assignment and gender role were evaluated in terms of psychological adjustment. Money and the Hampsons separated sex into three categories: biological sex characteristics, assigned sex or sex of rearing, and their newly added category, gender role. Gender role was how the child enacted their assigned sex and was not equivalent to our modern understanding of gender identity.[25] It was learned and shaped by "experiences encountered and transacted"—by living in one's assigned sex and being perceived as one's assigned sex. In their studies, they compared gender role with the other two sex categories and found that even in cases where sex of rearing did not match gonadal or chromosomal sex, it still matched the child's gender role. To make this argument, Money and the Hampsons had to find a way to assess children's gender role. In the course of their study, they developed their own mélange of psychological appraisals, consisting of interviews, observations of behavior, and psychological tests. They observed children and interviewed them to assess how they described themselves. Infants and small children, of course, could not be questioned, and often parents, who had their own understanding of their child's sex, stepped in as translators and observers of their children's gender role.

A roundtable discussion from 1954 shows the evolving application of the new gender role concept. The debate between Wilkins and his team at the Pediatric Endocrinology Clinic and a group of medical experts from Hospital of the University of Pennsylvania dealt with the particular tricky case of the doubtful sex of a nine-year-old girl called Geraldine. Her mother had brought her to University of Pennsylvania Hospital in July 1953 because (in the mother's words) she had a "growth on her privates."[26] During multiple examinations, physicians determined that the girl had "a testis, and a pretty good-sized phallus" as well as a "well-developed vagina which could be functional,"[27] a cervix, and a uterus.[28] Based on the presence of a testis, the doctors at the University of Pennsylvania Hospital determined that the girl was actually a boy and suggested the child be psychologically prepared for a change of sex. The mother, however, was strongly opposed to the plan. On the advice of Frank Fremont-Smith of the Josiah Macy Jr. Foundation, whose organization was also funding John Money's research position, Paul Györgi, chief of pediatrics at the Hospital of the University of Pennsylvania, sent Geraldine to the Johns Hopkins Hospital, where she was examined by Lawson Wilkins and gynecological surgeon Howard Jones. John Money and Joan Hampson also interviewed the child during her visit to the Johns Hopkins Hospital. At that time, Money and Hampson had already interviewed forty-four patients for their psychologic evaluation of hermaphroditic patients in the course of Wilkins's cortisone study, and they were in the process of getting their findings ready for publication.

Rather than determining which of Geraldine's sex characteristics pointed to her true sex, they assessed her gender role and whether it matched the sex she was growing up in. On January 21, 1954, both teams met in Philadelphia to discuss their findings at the interuniversity roundtable conference.[29] The experts at Hopkins had no doubt, testis or not, that Geraldine was a girl. In their assessment of her sex, her gonads did not matter as much as the gender role she assumed. "I am sure that by now it is abundantly evident that we at Hopkins do not put much weight in gonads per se," Hampson stated.[30] But if biology did not determine sex, how did the team from Johns Hopkins come to the conclusion that Geraldine was a girl? By assessing her gender role through observation and tests. Based on their encounters with the girl, they reported that her mannerisms—"posturing, gesturing, position of limbs when sitting and talking, inflection and rhythm of speech"—were entirely feminine after ten years of living as a girl. After a set of intelligence tests, Money and Hampson performed a thematic apperception test (TAT) to determine Geraldine's orientation as female or male. The TAT had been developed by Christiana D. Morgan and Henry A. Murray at Harvard University in 1935.[31] The idea behind this psychological test was that if subjects interpreted a complex situation, it revealed much about the person who was trying to make sense of it. During the test, participants were asked to interpret a set of ambiguous pictures and make up an oral or written story about them. Money used the tests to gain a fuller picture of how children positioned themselves as male or female and Geraldine "gave clear evidence in the TAT stories of a feminine orientation toward men."[32] Their assessment also included what they called "oblique" observations of play and behavior and interviews with Geraldine, again concluding that she "gave clear evidence in the TAT stories of a feminine orientation toward men."[33]

"Feminine orientation toward men" seemed to include a rather socially determined notion of female endangerment. Geraldine, Money observed, "unthinkingly regarded females as constantly in peril of being suddenly scared or assaulted by men," a reaction he credited to the girl's background with a violent and abusive father.[34] More significantly, she also "automatically placed herself in the female role while narrating the stories" and regarded herself as a girl.[35] During her assessment, she reacted to the multiple investigations of her gender role with her own assertion of herself as a female. When Money asked her, "If some blind person came to you and said: 'Are you a boy or a girl?' What would you say?" Geraldine replied that she knew that she "was part boy" but that she wouldn't tell him. Instead, "she would tell him she was a girl, she added."[36]

The experts from the University of Pennsylvania did not agree with the Hopkins assessment. First of all, Paul György thought it did matter that Geraldine had a testis. For him, the case was far from clear-cut. Accordingly, he and his colleagues had a divergent interpretation of Geraldine's behavior. For example, the girl wanted "a holster . . . two guns, a guitar, and a tie" for Christmas, and "her favorite television program [was] Gene Autry with a close second being Hopalong Cassidy."[37] In their opinion, this was clear evidence that her behavior and interests were male and that she was therefore a boy. There is now a vast body of critical scholarship that calls into question scientific studies where toy choice and play behavior are measured in normative gendered terms.[38] Yet even in 1954, toy choice shows that the terrain between masculinity and femininity was highly contested, and its meanings needed proper contextualization. Hampson argued that Geraldine's toy choice and play behavior were, quite on the contrary, evidence of her female gender role. After all, she had not just asked for "two guns and a holster," Hampson explained; she also wanted "a cowgirl suit to wear it on!" This exchange was far from trivial. Once Money and the Hampson detached sex from biology by arguing that a child's masculinity and femininity (or—to use their new term—gender role) was determined by the sex they were growing up in and not by hormones or sex chromosomes, they had to assess these qualities through social norms of male and female behavior.

The two groups might have disagreed about what constituted Geraldine's true sex, yet they all seemed to agree on what was the better sex for her: to remain a girl and become a woman. Even György settled with this assessment in the end, although for different reasons. For Money and Hampson, it was the accumulation of experiences that shaped the child's gender role, and their assessments of her gender role thus determined what was the right sex for Geraldine. Györgi disagreed but thought keeping Geraldine in the female sex was a pragmatic solution to a biological conundrum. Medical intervention contributed to no small amount; her testis had already been removed during her stay at Hopkins. That he thought she was really a boy but also believed that she could be raised as a girl is just one indicator of a fundamental shift toward privileging social functioning over what had long been considered biological truths.

In 1955, the same year Money and the Hampsons published the results of their three-and-a-half-year study in the *Bulletin of the Johns Hopkins Hospital*, Lawson Wilkins authored a paper in the September issue of *Pediatrics*, the official journal of the American Academy of Pediatrics.[39] Addressing an audience of pediatricians, he discussed questions of classification, diagnosis, and treatment in cases of hermaphroditism. At the forefront was the rather urgent (in his estimation) question of selection of sex in cases that he classified as "female pseudohermaphrodites with CAH" and in various forms of "intersexes." There was, Wilkins complained, "a lack of understanding of the principles by which the sex of rearing should be selected," and he hoped that providing physicians with "a better understanding" of these questions would aid them "to avoid some of the errors of the past."[40] His findings were based on the study of seventy cases at his Pediatric Endocrinology Clinic. Significantly, like Money and the Hampsons in their sister publications, he chose to differentiate between "sex of rearing" and biological aspects of sex.

The sex in which the child was raised was of extreme importance and had to be chosen wisely—that is, based on the realization of what was the best sex for the child and not "on the traditional belief that the sex chromosomal pattern, the gonads or the hormones which they produce are inevitably intrinsic determinants of an individual's psychosexual development and inclinations."[41] Since the ultimate goal of sex assignment was to ensure a well-adjusted child and eventually adult, the physician had to diagnose the child first in order to make a prognosis of sexual development. In cases of CAH, female genitals could look male, he warned, and parents and the uninformed practitioner might decide on the male sex for a female child. But once the diagnosis was made and with the newly established cortisone treatment, the child could be raised as a girl.

Wilkins's recommendations repeated Money and the Hampsons' conviction that gender role was acquired in the course of growing up and that for the children's gender role to match their sex of rearing and them to be well adjusted, their body, especially genitals, had to appear convincingly male or female. In the presence of informed physicians, the decision of the better sex in which to raise such children was to be based on the particular diagnosis of condition and the prognosis of somatic development. With cases of CAH, physicians knew that girls would look increasingly male and that with cortisone, this development could be altered and arrested. These girls could now live as girls, according to Wilkins, because they could fulfill their role as a woman.

In other cases, the prognosis was less clear-cut, and as he had already practiced in his clinic, Wilkins proposed to base the decision of what sex to assign on "the anatomy of the external genitalia, particularly the size of the phallus or the presence of a serviceable vagina, without regard to the type of gonad, the chromosomal pattern or the structure of the internal genital tract."[42] In order to acquire a male or female gender role, these children had to be accepted and treated as male or female, and genitals signified this in an important way. The decision of which sex to assign was, based on Money and the Hampsons' study, shaped not by genitals' link to a child's chromosomal and hormonal sex but to how much they lend themselves to be surgically altered to look convincingly male or female.

The correct size of phallus was contingent on and constitutive for sex choice. In this measurement, it was depicted as common sense "that unless there is a fairly well-developed phallus the patient cannot function as a male and will be subjected to constant humiliation and embarrassment throughout life."[43] There was no surgical procedure at the time that could alter genital appearance in male pseudohermaphrodites with a very small penis or "external genitalia of entirely female type" to resemble a male, and thus these children were thought best raised in the female sex. A phallus could also be deemed too large, for example, in cases of girls with CAH. "If the clitoris is enlarged sufficiently to attract attention and arouse the curiosity of other children or neighbors it is best to remove it," Wilkins recommended; he suggested postponing the decision concerning clitorectomy until the child was two to four years of age.[44]

All of these recommendations were presented in a language of compassion and care, had the implicated treatment goal of adjustment, and were supposedly supported by the numbers of clinical cases they had studied at Hopkins. They were also grounded in unquestioned assumptions about the importance of binary gender norms and the necessity of medical intervention. "It is tragic, and unnecessary, to condemn such patients to live as males without any masculine equipment," Wilkins wrote in 1955, when discussing sex assignment in male pseudohermaphrodites.[45] "It is a most pathetic sight to see these girls gradually become more and more virilized as time goes on," he had said about girls with CAH in a panel discussion in 1948, justifying his recommendation that they become male.[46] In 1955, he claimed to build on "substantial evidence" that these recommendations did not "lead to abnormalities in psychosexual orientation and development" by referring to the clinical data Money and the Hampsons had accumulated over the previous three years.[47] Their study had shown that "the gender in which a child is reared is the predominant factor in determining the future sexual orientation" (i.e., gender role).[48] A set of social markers such "hair cut, the style of clothing, the name and gender of personal pronouns applied, the toys and type of play, in addition to the anatomy of the external genitals are all important influences in establishing in early life the child's conviction as to whether he or she is a boy or a girl, provided there is not an attitude of confusion or uncertainty on the part of the parents,"[49] Wilkins wrote. Not biology but the consistent enactment and embodiment of their gender role was crucial for the children's conviction as to whether they were a boy or a girl.

Afterlife

Between the early 1950s and the early 1970s, the Hopkins findings were widely circulated and adapted as standard medical knowledge. Not surprisingly, clinician-researcher networks played an important role in how the Hopkins findings became standard medical knowledge. Starting in the late 1950s, the Hopkins findings were integrated into major pediatric textbooks, such as Luther Emmett Holt's classic *Diseases of Infancy and Childhood* and Waldo E. Nelson's *Pediatrics*.[50] The next generation of pediatric endocrinology textbooks, in the 1960s and 1970s, also incorporated aspects of the Hopkins findings. Not everything was taken up in the same way, though.[51]

Money and the Hampsons had made a bold pronouncement in their recommendations: that it might very well be the case that not only did children with intersex learn their gender role in the course of growing but that their clinical data produced evidence that their theory might apply to all humans. This particular idea was not taken up to its full extent by clinicians. Yet the idea of a "gender role" made an impressive career by itself. Reformulated as gender identity in the 1960s, it became a crucial term in psychology and the subsequent medical assessment of transgender. In the 1970s and 1980s, feminists started applying the idea of gender to argue that masculinity and femininity were culturally and socially constructed and could thus be relearned. In their discussions, they often referred back to the clinical evidence supposedly provided by the study of intersex children at Wilkins's Pediatric Endocrinology Clinic.[52]

The standardized recommendations of early sex assignment and genital surgery were uniformly accepted into practice and, as a vast body of scholarship has shown, applied unquestionably until the 1990s, when an emergent intersex patient movement called attention to the devastating consequences of invasive genital surgeries on mind and body.[53] Many activists, patients, and scholars also questioned the binary notion of sex into which intersex patients were forced and instead recommended a wait-and-see approach. Most intersex activists are still contesting the ongoing practice of surgically "correcting" genitals in infancy and are demanding legislation that would make these surgeries illegal before an age when consent is possible.[54]

Notes

1. This article is based on my findings in my forthcoming book *Making Gender* (Chicago: University of Chicago Press).
2. Some scholars have argued for expanding our categories of sex. See Anne Fausto-Sterling, "The Five Sexes: Why Male and Female Are Not Enough," *The Sciences*, March–April 1993, 20–24.
3. After much debate, a new terminology was introduced in the early twenty-first-century, namely "disorders of sexual development" (DSD), although not without controversy. On DSD, see Ellen K. Feder and Katrina Karkazis, "What's in a Name? The Controversy over 'Disorders of Sex Development,'" *Hastings Center Report* 38, no. 5 (2008): 33–36. Some have suggested the usage of the alternative term "divergence" or "difference of sexual development." See, for example, Elizabeth Reis, *Bodies in Doubt: An American History of Intersex* (Baltimore: Johns Hopkins University Press, 2009); Anne Fausto-Sterling, *Sexing the Body: Gender Politics and the Construction of Sexuality* (New York: Basic Books, 2000). In this chapter, I use the terms of my actors.
4. Hugh Hampton Young, *Genital Abnormalities: Hermaphroditism & Related Adrenal Diseases* (Baltimore: Williams & Wilkins, 1937).
5. On the study of hermaphroditism in nineteenth-century Europe, see Alice Domurat Dreger, *Hermaphrodites and the Medical Invention of Sex* (Cambridge, MA: Harvard University Press, 1998). On the United States, see Reis, *Bodies in Doubt*.
6. This rationale built on Klebs's classification schema in E. Klebs, *Handbuch Der Pathologischen Anatomie* (Berlin: Hirschwald, 1876).
7. See Geertje Mak, *Doubting Sex: Inscriptions, Bodies and Selves in Nineteenth-Century Hermaphrodite Case Histories* (Manchester: Manchester University Press, 2012).
8. On childbirth practices in the United States, see Charlotte G. Borst, *Catching Babies: The Professionalization of Childbirth, 1870–1920* (Cambridge, MA: Harvard University Press, 1995).
9. See, for example, Jacob E. Finesinger, Joe V. Meigs, and Hirsh W. Sulkowitch, "Clinical, Psychiatric and Psychoanalytic Study of a Case of Male Pseudohermaphroditism," *American Journal of Obstetrics and Gynecology* 44, no. 2 (1942): 310–17; F. M. Ingersoll and J. E. Finesinger, "A Case of Male Pseudohermaphroditism, the Importance of Psychiatry in the Surgery of This Condition," *Surgical Clinics of North America* 27 (1947): 1218–25.
10. In 1948, a new test developed by Murray Barr (The Barr Body Test) allowed clinicians to check for the second, inactive, X-chromosome. This added yet another (although at times unreliable) variable for sex to their expanding repertoire. See Fiona Alice Miller, "'Your True and Proper Gender': The Barr Body as a *Good Enough* Science of Sex," *Studies in History and Philosophy of Biological and Biomedical Sciences* 37 (2006): 449–83.

11. On the focus on sex, sex change, and rejuvenation in early endocrinology, see Chandak Sengoopta, *The Most Secret Quintessence of Life: Sex, Glands, and Hormones, 1850–1950* (Chicago: University of Chicago Press, 2006). On pediatric endocrinology, see Delbert A. Fisher, "A Short History of Pediatric Endocrinology in North America," *Pediatric Research* 55, no. 4 (2004): 716–26, 717–20.

12. Fisher, "A Short History of Pediatric Endocrinology in North America," 717.

13. Lawson Wilkins, *The Diagnosis and Treatment of Endocrine Disorders in Childhood and Adolescence* (Springfield, IL: Thomas, 1950). On Wilkins, see also C. J. Migeon, "Lawson Wilkins and My Life: Part 1," *International Journal of Pediatric Endocrinology* 2014, no. Suppl 1 (2014): S2; C. J. Migeon, "Lawson Wilkins and My Life: Part 2," *International Journal of Pediatric Endocrinology* 2014, no. Suppl 1 (2014): S3; C. J. Migeon, "Lawson Wilkins and My Life: Part 3," *International Journal of Pediatric Endocrinology* 2014, no. Suppl 1 (2014): S4.

14. For Wilkins's first case of adrenal hyperplasia, see L. Wilkins, W. Fleischmann, and J. E. Howard, "Macrogenitosomia Precox Associated with Hyperplasia of the Androgenic Tissue of the Adrenal and Death from Corticoadrenal Insufficiency," *Endocrinology* 26 (1940): 385–95; Lawson Wilkins and Curt P. Richter, "A Great Craving for Salt by a Child with Cortico-Adrenal Insufficiency," *JAMA* 114, no. 10 (1940): 866–68.

15. Although many women with CAH oppose this classification; Katrina Alicia Karkazis, *Fixing Sex: Intersex, Medical Authority, and Lived Experience* (Durham, NC: Duke University Press, 2008), 245.

16. For panel and participants, see A. W. Jacobsen et al., "The Adrenal Gland in Health and Disease," *Pediatrics* 3, no. 4 (1949): 515–48.

17. Jacobsen et al., 548.

18. See Sandra Eder, "The Birth of Gender: Clinical Encounters with Hermaphroditic Children at Johns Hopkins (1940–1956)" (Dissertation, Johns Hopkins University, 2011). On how social norms such as heterosexuality and marriage shaped medical decisions, see also Elizabeth Reis, *Bodies in Doubt: An American History of Intersex* (Baltimore: Johns Hopkins University Press, 2009), 82ff.

19. See Lawson Wilkins et al., "The Suppression of Androgen Secretion by Cortisone in a Case of Congenital Adrenal Hyperplasia," *Bulletin of the Johns Hopkins Hospital* 86 (1950): 249–52; L. Wilkins et al., "Treatment of Congenital Adrenal Hyperplasia with Cortisone," *Journal of Clinical Endocrinology* 11 (1951): 1–25.

20. John Money, "Hermaphroditism; an Inquiry into the Nature of a Human Paradox" (Dissertation, Harvard University, 1952).

21. John Money, Joan G. Hampson, and John L. Hampson, "An Examination of Some Basic Sexual Concepts: The Evidence of Human Hermaphroditism," *Bulletin of the Johns Hopkins Hospital* 97 (1955): 301–19, n. 303.

22. Money, Hampson, and Hampson, 308.

23. Money, Hampson, and Hampson.

24. See, for example, Suzanne J. Kessler, *Lessons from the Intersexed* (New Brunswick, NJ: Rutgers University Press, 1998); Fausto-Sterling, *Sexing the Body*; Katrina Alicia Karkazis, *Fixing Sex: Intersex, Medical Authority, and Lived Experience* (Durham, NC: Duke University Press, 2008); Ellen K. Feder, *Making Sense of Intersex: Changing Ethical Perspectives in Biomedicine* (Bloomington: Indiana University Press, 2014).

25. In 1964, Californian psychiatrist Robert Stoller introduced the term "gender identity" to describe the inner sense of knowing to which sex one belongs. See R. J. Stoller, "A Contribution to the Study of Gender Identity," *International Journal of Psychoanalysis* 45 (1964): 220–26.

26. P. Gyorgy et al., "Inter-University Round Table Conference by the Medical Faculties of the University of Pennsylvania and Johns Hopkins University. Psychological Aspects of the Sexual Orientation of the Child with Particular Reference to the Problem of Intersexuality," *Journal of Pediatrics* 47, no. 6 (1955): 771–90, p. 771.

27. Gyorgy et al., 779.

28. Gyorgy et al., 778.

29. Present at the roundtable were several pediatricians, psychologists, psychiatrists, a social worker, and the medical director of the Macy Foundation. The transcript of the meeting was published in the *Journal of Pediatrics* in 1955.

30. Gyorgy et al., "Inter-University Round Table Conference," 784.

31. Christiana D. Morgan and Henry A. Murray, "A Method for Investigating Fantasies: The Thematic Apperception Test," *Archives of Neurology and Psychiatry* 34, no. 2 (1935): 289–306.

32. Gyorgy et al., "Inter-University Round Table Conference," 782.

33. Gyorgy et al.

34. Gyorgy et al.

35. Gyorgy et al.

36. Gyorgy et al.

37. Gyorgy et al., 788.

38. See, for example, Rebecca M. Jordan-Young, *Brain Storm: The Flaws in the Science of Sex Differences* (Cambridge, MA: Harvard University Press, 2010); Anne Fausto-Sterling, *Myths of Gender: Biological Theories about Women and Men* (New York: Basic Books, 1985).

39. Lawson Wilkins et al., "Hermaphroditism: Classification, Diagnosis, Selection of Sex and Treatment," *Pediatrics* 16 (1955): 287–302.

40. Wilkins et al., 287.

41. Alison Redick, "American History XY: The Medical Treatment of Intersex, 1916–1955" (Dissertation, New York University, 2004), 287.

42. Wilkins et al., "Hermaphroditism," 296.

43. Wilkins et al. On phallus size as indicator of sex assignment, see Fausto-Sterling, *Sexing the Body*, 57–63.

44. Wilkins et al., "Hermaphroditism," 296.

45. Wilkins et al.

46. Jacobsen et al., "The Adrenal Gland in Health and Disease," 548.

47. Wilkins et al., "Hermaphroditism," 296.

48. Wilkins et al. At the time, "'sexual orientation' referred to one's subjective sense of maleness or femaleness, not to one's erotic preference for male versus female partners." See Rebecca M. Young, "Sexing the Brain: Measurement and Meaning in Biological Research on Human Sexuality" (Dissertation, Columbia University, 2000), n. 8, 200.

49. Wilkins et al., "Hermaphroditism," 296.

50. L. Emmett Holt, Rustin McIntosh, and L. Emmett Holt, *Holt Pediatrics*, 12th ed. (New York: Appleton-Century-Crofts, 1953); Waldo E. Nelson, ed., *Textbook of Pediatrics*, 7th ed. (Philadelphia: Saunders, 1959).

51. On the early transmission of the Hopkins recommendations, see Sandra Eder, "Gender and Cortisone: Clinical Practice and Transatlantic Exchange in the Medical Management of Intersex in the 1950s," *Bulletin of the History of Medicine* 92, no. 4 (2018): 604–33.

52. See, for example, Germaine Greer, *The Female Eunuch* (New York: McGraw-Hill, 1971); Ann Oakley, *Sex, Gender and Society: Towards a New Society* (London: Maurice Temple Smith Ltd., 1972). On gender's transformation, see Jennifer Germon, *Gender: A Genealogy of an Idea* (New York: Palgrave Macmillan, 2009).

53. To name just a few, see Kessler, *Lessons*; Alice Domurat Dreger, *Intersex in the Age of Ethics* (Hagerstown, MD: University Publishing Group, 1999); Alice D. Dreger, "Intersex and Human Rights: The Long View," in *Ethics and Intersex*, edited by Sharon E. Sytsma (Dordrecht, London: Springer, 2006), 73–86; I. A. Hughes et al., "Consensus Statement on Management of Intersex Disorders," *Archives of Disease in Childhood* 91, no. 7 (2006): 554–63; Karkazis, *Fixing Sex*; Morgan Holmes, *Critical Intersex: Queer Interventions* (Burlington, VT: Ashgate, 2009); Feder, *Making Sense of Intersex*; Zine Magubane, "Spectacles and Scholarship: Caster Semenya, Intersex Studies, and the Problem of Race in Feminist Theory," *Signs* 39, no. 3 (2014): 761–85.

54. In California, a legislative initiative (SB201) to bar doctors from performing "treatment or intervention on the sex characteristics of a person born with variations in their physical sex characteristics who is under 6 years of age unless the treatment or intervention is medically necessary" was rejected in January 2020. https://leginfo. legislature.ca.gov/faces/billTextClient.xhtml?bill_id=201920200SB201 (accessed February 17, 2020). Elizabeth Reis notes that CAH has become a notable exception in this rejection of surgery. CARES, a large parent organization dedicated to the treatment and support of children with CAH, considers it a separate condition and rejects subsuming it under the DSD/intersex umbrella. CARES also opposes a ban on early nonconsensual genital surgery, maintaining that these interventions are "medical necessary" (defined loosely also in terms of psychological health) or, if not necessary in the strictest sense, then at least beneficial and desirable. On the conflict between CAH and DSD/intersex, see Elizabeth Reis, *Bodies in Doubt: An American History of Intersex*, 2nd ed. (Baltimore: Johns Hopkins University Press, forthcoming 2021).

Chapter 5

Depathologizing Trans Childhood

The Role of History in the Clinic

JULES GILL-PETERSON

The first time I experienced medical gatekeeping, I was entirely unprepared for how painful it would feel. I needed to meet with a psychiatrist to acquire a letter justifying a request for insurance coverage of electrolysis. This was hardly my first encounter with the *idea* of the diagnostic model of gender dysphoria, or the pathologization of trans identity it so often sparks. But it was my first time being asked to give an account of myself that fit the medical biography of a trans woman. Although my employer's health plan's marketing campaigns around trans health care assured me that it had adopted a gender-affirmative care model and was expanding its welcoming access, the continuing categorization of facial hair removal as elective meant that I needed a psychiatrist to verify my adherence to *DSM-V* criteria.

In my first appointment, when the psychiatrist asked what I did for a living, I explained that I was a university professor working in the field of transgender studies and that I had recently published a book on the history of trans medicalization. I was relieved when this elicited a smile: *Well*, the psychiatrist said, dropping the fourth wall, *I guess, in a way, you know more about this process than I do.* I was happy to be invited to treat the sessions and the letter as a strategic exercise, a way to access care that I knew I needed. I had become *interesting*, and it felt like this session was not an evaluative process to determine if I was "trans enough" to not have to pay out-of-pocket for electrolysis. The psychiatrist asked questions; I offered honest answers. It seemed to go well. At the end of two sessions, he assured me that I had provided more than enough material and that my life was compelling. At one point during a story I told about my childhood, which I thought was unremarkable, he began to cry.

After the sessions, I waited, anxiously, for an update on my letter. Weeks passed, then months. I was extremely busy otherwise: my first book had just come out, I was conducting new research on a fellowship, and I had a series of lectures booked around the country. After nearly four months of silence, I finally registered how much time had passed and contacted the psychiatrist. He told me he had not written my letter and that he was feeling "anxious" about it because he was not sure that I really fit the *DSM* criteria for gender dysphoria. Perhaps, he suggested, I should wait until my transition was more convincingly "trans female" and then we could try again.

I was devastated. Not only was the delay amplifying my dysphoria, but I also felt betrayed. I thought I had been invited to treat the diagnostic and pathologizing dimensions of this process for what they were: arbitrary and undesirable, if nevertheless obligatory. The psychiatrist had given me an "in" by recognizing *my* expertise as a scholar of transgender studies. Or so I thought. It would take several more months, several hundred dollars in fees, and a far more scripted account of myself to convince him to write the letter. When I finally read it, I felt sad. It did not seem to describe me at all.

I begin with this story in a chapter about trans children because I was *not* a child when this gatekeeping happened. I was in my thirties. Despite a PhD and a published book on the history of transgender medicine, I found myself at the mercy of a single clinician whose ambivalence about my conformity to the *DSM* was delaying not my actual electrolysis treatment but the simple ability *to request access* to it. (Later, I found out that the health plan most likely would *not* cover it, after all.) All of this occurred under the auspices of a gender-affirmative care model that has come to be seen as the best practice in trans health care in recent years. Despite my academic knowledge about medicalization, the psychiatrist's recognition of it, and an explicitly stated commitment to gender-affirmative care, I experienced the emotional and material fallout of being pathologized as not trans enough, with the gatekeeping it often enables. Having had this experience as an adult, quick on the heels of finishing a book about the history of transgender children, I felt a longstanding question with new sharpness: *If I'm having this much trouble, how on earth do trans kids manage to get competent health care?*

Drawing on this scene of gatekeeping and the research informing that book, *Histories of the Transgender Child*, this chapter explores the history of transgender children's medicalization during the twentieth century to ask some difficult questions of the present-day pediatric clinic. While the mechanics of evaluation, gatekeeping, pathologization, and normalization in pediatric trans medicine have been detailed by a number of scholars, a historical lens contributes a different insight.[1] I contextualize how the ongoing pathologization of trans childhood is rooted in a history where sex and gender were identified by medical science with children's *plasticity*. While the wane of reparative and conversion treatment models today signals a major improvement for trans young people and adults alike, the continued centrality of plasticity to the medical model maintains a deep-rooted level of pathologization: childhood itself is equated with the etiology of gender. Childhood is understood to be the process through which gender in general and transness in particular emerge and, thereby, the process through which transition finds its foothold in the growing body. Working toward gender justice and self-determination for children today involves a clinical reckoning with the historical inheritance of plasticity, for it carries an easily overlooked racial history that actively limits the ability of clinicians to provide meaningfully affirmative and equitable care.

How Childhood Became the Etiology of Gender

The opening of the Gender Identity Clinic at the Johns Hopkins Hospital in November 1966 was seen at the time as a watershed moment for the new field of transgender medicine, then called transsexual medicine. Patients began working their way through the clinic's paradigmatic tiered process, which included extensive medical and psychiatric examination, hormone therapy, and the requirement of living publicly in one's gender identity for at least a year before surgery.[2] By providing gender affirmation surgery after several decades during which the United States lagged behind other countries in this field, the Hopkins clinic has been regarded as an important first in U.S. transgender history and medicine.[3] What prefaces the opening of the clinic, however, challenges that historical narrative. At the end of 1964, over a year earlier, psychologist John Money and several of his colleagues had been aggressively lobbying to take on as a full-time patient someone they had recently diagnosed as transsexual. In January 1965, they succeeded: the Criminal Court for Baltimore City, where this prospective patient was on trial for burglary, issued a court order for "surgical sex repair" at Hopkins in lieu of a jail sentence.[4] The judge apparently agreed with Money that the defendant's criminal record was best understood as a kind of side effect of what the court documents named "transsexualism" and that surgery would end their frequent arrest and institutionalization by the state. This patient, who I will refer to by the initials "G.L.," was moved from jail to the hospital. They key detail is that G.L. was only seventeen years old. Their mother provided written consent to the court order, as well as for the surgery.[5] Money and other clinicians involved had actually known G.L. since they were thirteen years old, when G.L.'s school had contacted Hopkins for advice on how to control G.L.'s behavior. What G.L.'s case indicates is that the first sanctioned gender confirmation surgery at Hopkins was arranged for a child. However, the surgery never took place. Faculty—primarily psychiatrists who disapproved of offering any surgical procedures for a condition they considered psychological— managed to delay the surgery several times. Although G.L.'s motives remain unknown, during this period, they ran away from the hospital and were never heard from again.

Why does it matter for transgender medicine that this "watershed" moment is prefaced by a child? G.L.'s case illustrates the double bind in which children found themselves as the medical model took shape during the second half of the twentieth century. On the one hand, something about their developing bodies was prized as essential to clinicians and researchers aiming to develop reliable techniques for transition and gender reassignment. On the other hand, they were also meant to completely disappear as people, erased by the institutions and discourses that comprised the medical model. In some cases, like G.L.'s, transgender children found doctors who were willing to oversee hormones, social transition, and even gender confirmation surgery under the pretense of clinical research. For many other children, by contrast, clinicians were more interested in trying to extinguish trans identity during childhood because they theorized it as the developmental period of its onset. These latter clinics tended to favor psychotherapy or psychoanalysis over medical transition.[6]

Both clinical approaches shared an underlying principle: the plasticity of gender. Today, the most recognized area of this research concerns neuroplasticity, the capacity of the brain to adapt and change over time in response to environmental input. A range of efforts involving brain imaging scans are attempting to isolate what a "male" or "female" brain looks like or how the brains of transgender people supposedly correspond to the morphology associated with cisgender people of their gender identity rather than their assigned sex at birth.[7] However, during the twentieth century, it was not the brain but the endocrine system that received the most attention. In *Histories of the Transgender Child*, I treat this history of gender's plasticity at far greater length, but what follows specifies its most crucial aspects in order to interpret the significance of G.L.'s admission to Hopkins in 1965 and what its legacy remains in today's clinic.

For the first half of the twentieth century, both endocrinology and the medical and psychiatric fields that dealt with human sex did not employ a particularly robust concept of a male/female binary. Instead, researchers and clinicians worked from the hypothesis that "sex" was definitionally what they termed "bisexual," which is to say *normally* a mix of male and female. The idea was first anchored in endocrine experiments in changing the sex of animals, mostly via gonad transplantation.[8] This apparent capacity to change sex in animals also took on a developmental contour, which allowed biologists and endocrinologists to argue that all human life started out, in utero, with the biological potential to become both sexes. While the course of human development led to one sex becoming predominant, this view held that humans never lost the potential to "become" the other sex.[9] Children were conceptually vital to this discourse, as child development became the strongest case for scientists and clinical researchers to show *how*, as human beings grow, their sex undergoes changes that, by the end of puberty or adulthood, generally result in a mostly binary-looking sex.[10] The principle underlining this wide field of biological and medical research was plasticity: the concept that human form, biological and psychological, is qualitatively plastic, that it changes as it grows, both endogenously and due to outside intervention.

Childhood, crucially, was identified as the most plastic period in human life, and so children were of interest to the new field of transgender medicine by the 1960s because they seemed to incarnate a kind of proof of plasticity. At the same time, doctors hoped that transgender children might offer clinical opportunities to actually experiment on plasticity during childhood in order to standardize techniques for medically altering human sex. By the mid-1960s, when transgender medicine was becoming an established field, clinical researchers had been partially successful in this endeavor, although up to that point, their research was conducted not with transgender children but with intersex children. The new thesis of the plasticity of sex during development had radically reframed the old concept of "hermaphroditism," which had long been considered a kind of pathological difference in kind from binary sex.[11] Researchers instead began to wonder if the plasticity they now assumed informed all sexual differentiation might also account for the nonbinary embodiment of intersex infants and children while also providing a material foothold for encouraging or imposing a normative development trajectory. Despite the fact that most intersex conditions carry no medical risks, doctors and endocrinologists began to construe nonnormative genitals or endocrine organs as necessitating correction toward a binary form.[12]

Research hospitals like Johns Hopkins developed the initial techniques for surgical alteration of the sexed body through attempts to produce the binary-looking genitals and secondary sex characteristics they felt intersex infants and children ought to have. At Hopkins, surgeon Hugh Hampton Young performed procedures that were often incredibly painful and included dangerous complications on very young children. Although he obtained the consent of parents, such surgeries were typically carried out without informing his child patients of the reason (or before they were old enough to be informed). And in their obsessive aesthetic focus on producing the sex binary, these methods for influencing intersex plasticity rarely resulted in any therapeutic benefit.[13] In the 1940s, this clinical research also began to include new synthetic hormone therapies. By midcentury, many of the resulting experimental techniques for influencing the plasticity of sex during childhood development were transferred and remade for transgender medicine.[14] And in this context, children like G.L. were of immense experimental value because of the living plasticity of their gender. In short, because of transgender medicine's technical and conceptual reliance on plasticity to alter sex and gender, children were the invisible bedrock of the medical model at the time of its formation. Children's bodies granted the closest thing to real access to gender's plasticity, and so the history of trans medicine is in many ways a shadow history of children. This was the process by which childhood was equated with the etiology of transgender identity, specifically, but also gender identity in general.

Plasticity is also a racialized concept, albeit in a highly abstract manner. Plasticity is, strictly speaking, invisible: it cannot be imaged under a microscope as a "part" of the body, although its effects can be observed and influenced in the living body. As an idea, then, plasticity needed something to make it cohere as it was shaping the field of endocrinology: an image, metaphor, or sibling concept that could lend it legibility. I argue that plasticity was equated by scientists and clinical researchers with an abstract form of whiteness to give it a more tangible form. The equivalence was built around the implicit idea that being malleable *and* receptive to normalization are qualities correspondent to white bodies. Far from an obvious association, the whiteness of plasticity was carefully constructed over decades through the explicit politics of eugenics that governed the life sciences in the first half of the twentieth century, as well as serving more specifically as an alibi for painful and medically unnecessary surgery on white intersex children presented as a "humane" endeavor to produce normality.[15] In this sense, plasticity was racialized white, likewise, to justify the attention that white transgender and gender-nonconforming children received from the first generation of clinicians in transgender medicine at institutions like Hopkins. In construing white children as abnormal but potentially redeemable if they were to submit to normalization, these clinicians laid the groundwork for the most rigid gatekeeping whose effects still linger today. The equation of plasticity with whiteness also explains how the medical model built in an implicit rejection of Black trans and other trans children of color, who were frequently turned away from clinics or willfully misdiagnosed by doctors and psychologists as homosexual or schizophrenic, more often sent to psychiatric wards or other carceral institutions because their blackness and brownness were read as *not plastic enough* for this new medical model.[16]

Conceiving of gender as intrinsically plastic enough to clinically manage transition, then, came at a high price for transgender children. The equation of gender's plasticity with childhood made children more often than not of abstract *research* interest to clinicians, rather than seeing them as human beings who deserved competent health care. The implicit racial logic buried in the concept of plasticity also began to stratify transgender health care for children and adults alike, compounding the existing racial disparities in U.S. health care that resulted in a situation that persists to the present day, where Black trans and transgender people of color still disproportionately lack access to safe and competent care.

Plasticity and Affirmative Care

Considering that the history of medicalization outlined above is defined by systematic efforts to erase trans identity and exclude as many people from health care as possible through extremely narrow diagnostic eligibility, the emergence of an affirmative care model in recent years is incredibly significant. And it has particularly positive consequences for children. The affirmative care model in pediatric transgender medicine is designed to give up the primary problem that had dogged children and young people's access to care in the past. The concern of clinicians is no longer to establish *if* a patient "really is trans" or not. Or, more precisely, the clinical role is no longer to assess whether or not a child will grow up to be transgender. Instead, the role of clinicians is to support and offer guidance to trans children and their families in whatever form each child feels concurs with their expressed gender identity, understanding that this may also change over time. In other words, affirmative care is meant to do just as its name implies: *affirm* the identities and wishes of trans people, rather than use medicalization to evaluate who counts as transgender and how medical support can be distributed on that basis.

The affirmative care model is, however, mostly an aspiration. In pediatric care, in particular, the model is primarily derived from several statements of principle. The World Professional Association for Transgender Health's *Standards of Care for the Health of Transsexual, Transgender, and Gender Nonconforming People* is frequently cited as one of the foundational documents.[17] These standards of care date from 2012, which makes them somewhat "old" in a rapidly expanding field of health care. More recently, in September 2018, the American Academy of Pediatrics (AAP) issued a statement on affirmative health care for trans children. That statement summarizes gender-affirmative care as that which "offer[s] developmentally appropriate care that is oriented toward understanding and appreciating the youth's gender experience. A strong, nonjudgmental partnership with youth and their families can facilitate exploration of complicated emotions and gender-diverse expressions while allowing concerns to be raised in a supportive environment."[18] At the clinical level, the AAP model stresses a holistic, integrative approach that makes mental and physical health providers available as a team to collaborate with the children and their families.

The key phrase in this statement is "developmentally appropriate." It holds a contradiction that, in its widest aperture, questions whether or not "affirmative" care is even possible for children. Given that today's medical model continues to ground the delivery of care on the presumption that children are defined by their development, it is structured by the belief that they cannot be adequately autonomous or self-aware of their gendered growth but instead require some direction and management from adults. In this situation, much of the impact of the word "affirmative" is undercut. For instance, the authority of parents over their children's gender expression has, if unintentionally, been somewhat *magnified* by the affirmative care model, as it requires parents to be heavily involved in observing and interpreting their child's identity and behavior. The general outcome of this developmental logic has increased the vectors of governance bearing on transgender children through affirmative care, pulling them more tightly into the authority of medicalization. What's more, given that the affirmative care model is mostly an ideal, only the tiniest fraction of trans young people who might seek out affirmative care have the money, time, parental support, or other means to access it. Trans children living in poverty, trans children of color, trans children without supportive families, and trans children who experience other forms of marginalization are effectively shut out of this model of health care.[19] They barely even register in the outrageous antitrans public "debates" and attacks on trans children that are raging in North America and the United Kingdom.

Perhaps more important, however, the affirmative care model—quite ironically—can do relatively little to reduce the root pathologization of transgender children. To understand how that is the case, history has an active role to play in today's clinic. Childhood itself has been equated with the etiology of transness by medicine over the past century, as medical science and popular wisdom alike have come to imagine that gender identity takes form during childhood and that childhood itself is the plastic process—at once biological, cultural, and social—through which identity and embodiment cohere and establish their relationship as sex and gender. In this broader historical context, the expansion of health care into the lives of transgender children without accounting for the history of its reliance on the concept of plasticity only increases the conceptual association of childhood with pathogenesis.

The term "pathologization" registers here in a number of senses. First, there is the most literal clinical pathologization of transgender people in the medical setting. In its current form, the *DSM-V* diagnosis "gender dysphoria" technically does not pathologize transgender identity per se, but in practical usage and in effect, it continues to pathologize by requiring transgender people to seek some form of psychiatric supervision to access certain forms of medical transition.[20] Pathologization also bears a cultural significance that takes the form of trans-exceptionalization: outsourcing all of the instability of the gender binary onto transgender people when cisgender people do not have to justify how they know what their gender is, what their gender's etiology is, or why they might want access to health care or legal and social recognition of their gender's mere *existence*. And finally, in the case of children, childhood has been equated, because of its plasticity, with the etiology of transness in particular and gender identity in general, so that being a trans child is itself associated with pathology. Or, put differently, trans childhood is treated *conceptually* as a site of pathogenesis by medicine. This is best understood as a discursive feature of the medical model, one that is inherited from the era in which G.L. visited Hopkins, and so it remains implicitly active even when individual clinicians do not see trans identity as pathology or when they follow the affirmative care model.

Conclusion: Depathologization, Obsolescence, and Justice

Transgender people have long pursued *de*pathologization to imagine an end to pathologizing models, protocols, and discourses. As Amets Suess, Karine Espineira, and Pau Crego Walters explain in a 2014 article in *Transgender Studies Quarterly*, "The trans depathologization framework introduces a paradigm shift in the conceptualization of gender identities. From conceiving of gender transition as a mental disorder to recognizing it as a human right and expression of human diversity. From this perspective," they write, "the conflict is not situated in the individual trans person but in a society characterized by transphobia and gender binarism."[21] There are uniquely high stakes for children in making that shift because the individualization of conflict over gender in the transgender body has been disproportionately the experience of trans kids, whose developmental trajectories are fixated upon as *the* process through which transness is generated and, therefore, can be managed, affirmatively or otherwise. Add to this that gender self-determination for children and young people faces a unique set of barriers in the fact that Western culture does not grant children full civil rights, let alone the agency of self-determination. On the contrary, the law and cultural norms forcibly render children dependent and deprived of the ability to consent, to speak for themselves, and to represent their own interests, whether bodily, medical, legal, or economic. This situation hits transgender children and young people even harder in the form of legal barriers, such as the medical age of consent, but also in cultural attitudes that allow adults to say children are "too young" to know they are trans, that they might "grow out of it," or that their decisions to socially transition, take puberty blockers, or change their names are too complex for them to make.

In other words, I am arguing that the deep-rooted developmentalism and pathologization of transgender medicine forged in the middle decades of the twentieth century cannot be extinguished by the affirmative care model, at least in the case of children. This is because the delivery of pediatric care continues to rely on the conceptual and material affordances of gender's plasticity, which makes childhood into *the moment* when gender identity forms, as opposed to a moment in which transness can be greeted and affirmed as both real and desirable. The history of medicalization bears down on today's clinic in this way but from both sides. Transgender people, including children and youth, bring the weight of this history of pathologization, gatekeeping, and harm with them into the clinic, acutely aware that many before them have been forced to endure great pain, suffering, and interference with their access to competent care.[22] Clinicians, inheriting a model of gender's plasticity formed in the mid-twentieth century, cannot overcome this history on an individual level any more than individual trans people can. This was, in one sense, one of the lessons I learned when I experienced gatekeeping around my letter for electrolysis. No amount of knowledge granted by a PhD or my own research in trans medicalization could overcome my structural vulnerability to a system of evaluation that judged my gender as insufficiently normative. And if I could not protect myself from being pathologized, how could an eight-year-old or a sixteen-year-old child protect themselves?

What, then, can clinicians do differently in light of the history of transgender children? Change on the level of depathologization is slow. The violent arithmetic of trans youth suicidality, exposure to violence, and particularly the extreme levels of murder and hate crimes against Black trans women and trans women of color communities necessitates forms of harm reduction in the interim. While standards of affirmative care continue to be implemented, clinicians can work to educate themselves on the history of trans medicine, to acquaint themselves with this particular history of plasticity that bears down on trans children. Clinicians can also benefit from being candid about the mechanics of medicalization and the limitations of existing frameworks for care.

Admitting to young people in the clinic that they do not have all the answers or are able to override all the forms of harm embedded in the medical model opens a window for a dialogue about the possibility and limits of agency and self-determination.

I end *Histories of the Transgender Child* by suggesting that all adults, including clinicians, have scarcely imagined the tectonic shift that would be accomplished by actually *listening* to trans children's wishes, desires, and hopes. I still believe this, but I am also uncertain that clinicians can mitigate the harms of medicalization and pathologization through listening and affirmation alone. The clinical professionals involved in the delivery of pediatric trans medicine need to critically reflect on how to also take responsibility for the histories of pathologization, violence, gatekeeping, and harm that they inherit, if not only in medical concepts and techniques, then in the collective memory of the trans community. This was what was missing, after all, in my encounter with the psychiatrist writing my letter. He *did* recognize my expertise, both in my own gender identity and in the area of trans studies, but he did not demonstrate self-reflexivity about his immense power to determine the fate of my request for insurance coverage—not to mention its timing and likelihood of success. When he hesitated in writing my letter for several months because of his own anxiety—however sincere that was—he abdicated his responsibility in delivering care to me, as if forcing me to wait while experiencing dysphoria, with no indication why, were not a form of harm in and of itself. I choose to believe, out of personal experience as much as historical research, that a future where transness is not medicalized, and health care is available upon demand without prohibitive cost, is a future in which trans people of all ages will finally be free from a certain form of subjection we have carried for far too long. Until that day comes, clinicians have a responsibility to hold themselves accountable for what their profession has done in the past, as well as the immense power they continue to wield to this day, affirmative or otherwise. Difficult as it may be, perhaps the *only* ethical position for a clinician in pediatric trans medicine to hold is an avowed commitment to bringing about the obsolescence of their own position: to actively work in their profession toward ending the pathologization of trans children and young people altogether.

Notes

1. See Ann Travers, *The Trans Generation: How Trans Kids (and Their Parents) Are Creating a Gender Revolution* (New York: NYU Press, 2018); Claudia Castaneda, "Developing Gender: The Medical Treatment of Transgender Young People," *Social Science and Medicine* 143 (October 2015): 262–70; Tey Meadow, *Trans Kids: Being Gendered in the Twenty-First Century* (Berkeley: University of California Press, 2018).

2. John Money to Ram. W. Rapoport, August 2, 1973, Box 7, John Money Collection, Kinsey Institute, Bloomington, Indiana.

3. See Joanne Meyerowitz, *How Sex Changed: A History of Transsexuality in the United States* (Cambridge, MA: Harvard University Press, 2004); Susan Stryker, *Transgender History* (Berkeley, CA: Seal Press, 2008); Bernice Hausman, *Changing Sex: Transsexualism, Technology, and the Idea of Gender* (Durham, NC: Duke University Press, 1995).

4. *State of Maryland v. [G.L.]*, Indictment #1531 Y, January 5, 1965, Maryland State Archives.

5. I use plural pronouns to refer to G. L. to avoid assigning them any gender in the absence of a clear, expressed identity from them in the archive. I use the initials "G. L." because John Money included them in the one publication about G. L. from his career. See John Money and Florence Schwarz, "Public Opinion and Social Issues in Transsexualism: A Case Study in Medical Sociology," in *Transsexualism and Sex Reassignment*, ed. Richard Green and John Money (Baltimore: Johns Hopkins University Press, 1969), 255–70.

6. One contemporaneous clinic that espoused this kind of conversion therapy model was the University of California, Los Angeles Gender Clinic run by psychiatrist and psychoanalyst Robert Stoller. I discuss this clinic at length in *Histories of the Transgender Child* (Minneapolis: University of Minnesota Press, 2018), 143–50.

7. On the so-called gendered brain in neuroscience, see Rebecca Jordan-Young, *Brain Storm: The Flaws in the Science of Sex Difference* (Cambridge, MA: Harvard University Press, 2011).

8. In Europe, this research was made especially popular by Eugen Steinach, an endocrinologist who attempted to develop medical procedures for promoting the ideal health of human sex out of his experiments on the sexual plasticity of rats and guinea pigs. Eugen Steinach, *Sex and Life: Forty Years of Biological and Medical Experiments*, trans. Josef Loebel (New York: Viking Press, 1940). In the United States, the biologist Oscar Riddle likewise worked to transform the sex of birds, especially pigeons, via their endocrine systems. See Oscar Riddle, "A Case of Complete Sex-Reversal in the Adult Pigeon," *American Naturalist* 58, no. 655 (1924): 167–81.

9. One of the landmark experiments to establish that plasticity was developmental occurred in 1892 when Hans Driesch artificially cut a sea urchin embryo in half. When that embryo began to grow into two identical organisms, each roughly half the size of a normal embryo, Driesch interpreted that the plasticity of the embryo allowed it to adapt and reform itself in response to environmental pressure, affecting its eventual form. Hans Driesch, "The Potency of the First Two Cleavage Cells in Echinoderm Development: Experimental Production of Partial and Double Formations," in *Foundations of Experimental Endocrinology*, ed. Benjamin H. Willer and Jane M. Oppenheimer (Englewood Cliffs, NJ: Prentice Hall, 1964), 39–42. Endocrinologists like Steinach analogized from this cellular view to the human life span via childhood. See *Sex and Life*, 45–46.

10. An emblematic account of this leap from developmental plasticity to child development via the interdisciplinary field of the life sciences can be found in psychologist G. Stanley Hall's *Adolescence: Its Psychology and Its Relations to Physiology, Anthropology, Sociology, Sex, Crime, Religion, and Education* (New York: D. Appleton, 1904).

11. On the discursive shift from "hermaphroditism" to "intersex," see David A. Rubin, *Intersex Matters: Biomedical Embodiment, Gender Regulation, and Transnational Activism* (Albany: State University of New York Press, 2017), 21–48.

12. Intersex studies has critically detailed this process by which human diversity and variation in sexed embodiment has become construed as requiring medical intervention. See Georgiann Davis, *Contesting Intersex: The Dubious Diagnosis* (New York: New York University Press, 2015).

13. Young detailed a large collection of these cases in a textbook. See Hugh Hampton Young, *Genital Abnormalities, Hermaphroditism, and Related Adrenal Diseases* (Baltimore: Williams & Wilkins, 1937). However, his case study summaries rarely mention the impacts of his surgical protocols or admit their destructive and painful impact (except in passing). Those aspects of this history, from the perspectives of his patients, are found in medical records at Hopkins. Strict privacy regulations and federal law limit access to these records, which is why I cannot cite them in detail here; the relevant collection is the "Hermaphroditism" patient files of the Brady Urological Institute Records, at the Alan Chesney Mason Archives of the Johns Hopkins Hospital, Baltimore.

14. This is evident in the medical records of the Brady Urological Institute, where the same clinicians who worked with intersex children began to interact with potential transgender patients in the 1940s, evaluating whether or not to offer them similar surgical and hormonal procedures. These medical records are indexed under "Transvestism" and, later, "Transsexualism," Brady Urological Institute Records, at the Alan Chesney Mason Archives of the Johns Hopkins Hospital, Baltimore. Because strict privacy guidelines and federal law govern access to these records, I cannot cite any of them in detail here.

15. This relation between whiteness, medical violence, and humaneness is examined especially well in Iain Morland, "Gender, Genitals, and the Meaning of Being Human," in *Fuckology: Critical Essays on John Money's Diagnostic Concepts*, ed. Iain Morland and Nikki Sullivan (Chicago: University of Chicago Press, 2014), 69–100.

16. For a longer treatment of this convergence of racial logics, see Julian Gill-Peterson, "Trans of Color Critique Before Transsexuality," *Transgender Studies Quarterly* 5, no. 4 (2018): 606–20.

17. The World Professional Association for Transgender Health, *Standards of Care for the Health of Transsexual, Transgender, and Gender Nonconforming People, 7th Version* (WPATH, 2012).

18. Jason Rafferty, "Ensuring Comprehensive Care and Support for Transgender and Gender-Diverse Children and Adolescents," *Pediatrics* 142, no. 4 (September 2018), https://pediatrics.aappublications.org/content/142/4/e20182162.

19. For an extended discussion of these problems, see Travers, *The Trans Generation*.

20. American Psychiatric Association, "Gender Dysphoria," https://www.psychiatry.org/File%20Library/Psychiatrists/Practice/DSM/APA_DSM-5-Gender-Dysphoria.pdf.

21. Amets Suess, Karine Espineira, and Pau Crego Walters, "Depathologization," *Transgender Studies Quarterly* 1, no. 1 (2014): 74.

22. See Kate Eldridge, "'We Know Who We Are': Centering Queer and Trans Youth Narratives in the Move toward Affirmative Healthcare" (BPhil Honors Thesis, University of Pittsburgh, 2019).

Chapter 6

Race and Gender in the NICU

Wimpy White Boys and Strong Black Girls

CHRISTINE H. MORTON, KRISTA SIGURDSON, AND JOCHEN PROFIT

One of us first heard of "wimpy white boys" in the context of prematurity when we overheard a former neonatal nurse reassuring a coworker that her baby would be fine, even if she gave birth prematurely. "Black baby girls are really strong," she asserted forcefully. "I'm not going to worry about you." When asked about the basis for her positivity, she explained there was a concept called "wimpy white boy syndrome" (WWBS), which referred to clinical situations in the neonatal intensive care unit (NICU) in which white boys had the worst outcomes while Black girls had the best.

Neonatology is the branch of medicine concerned with the treatment and care of newborn babies. Neonatology physicians and neonatal nurses—herein referred to as neonatal clinicians—are trained specifically to handle the most complex and high-risk situations, which often stem from birth defects, preterm birth, or very low birthweight. It turns out that "if you've been doing this longer than a minute, you've probably heard" about wimpy white boy syndrome, as one neonatologist we spoke with affirmed; they added that "it's an observation that people have made, and you can walk from NICU to NICU to NICU, no matter where you are, and say that, and they will understand what that means. But yet, the fact that no one has put it on down on paper says there's something else there, too."[1]

We were curious about what this "something else" might be. Our interdisciplinary research team, composed of medical sociologists and neonatologists, develops measures for NICU quality of care and identifies racial/ethnic disparities. Recently, we published a systematic review of the literature on NICU quality of care in which we showed that the majority of studies indicate that nonwhite infants experience worse quality of neonatal care.[2] We were interested in how the "wimpy white boy" and the "strong Black girl" memes embedded in clinical contexts coexisted with evidence showing lower quality of care for Black infants. In a response to our systematic review, Dr. Wanda Barfield, director of the Division of Reproductive Health at the Centers for Disease Control and Prevention, affirmed the notion that cultural ideas about race affect quality and outcomes. She challenged clinicians to "dispel the myths of an inherent advantage by African American premature infants. The perception that an individual infant may have an advantage of survival on the basis of population measures does a disservice to that individual patient and may bias the care delivered."[3]

In this essay, we present a social, exploratory history of the wimpy white boy syndrome meme in perinatal care and problematize underlying meanings of its use in scientific, clinical, and informal discourses. We also critically illustrate how epidemiological-sociocultural concepts of race and gender may influence NICU care, NICU culture, and how parents perceive the care their babies receive. We consider the historical and cultural meanings of such phrases as "wimp" and "strong" and their connection to contemporary understanding of these terms as applied to premature infants and adults: what does it mean to be a wimpy male? Or a strong Black female? What are the connections between the clinical idea of WWBS in the NICU and other racialized and gendered concepts that circulate in society?

We reviewed scientific literature and conducted interviews by telephone or videoconference with American neonatal nurses, nurse practitioners, and physicians in the spring and summer of 2019. Our interviewees included men, women, white, Black, and U.S.- and foreign-born and trained clinicians. Because we promised clinicians anonymity and confidentiality, we do not note their names or individual characteristics when quoting them. We also read parent discussion board conversations about wimpy white boy syndrome by fifty-eight individual posters, whose gender and race were not noted, on the parenting websites BabyCenter.com and TheBump.com.[4]

Ideas about Race and Sex in Health Care Settings

The phrase "wimpy white boy syndrome" and the underlying idea of "wimpy white boys" juxtaposed against "strong Black girls" struck us as a jarring instance of racialized medicine at a time when maternal and infant health indicators are worsening, and the emergence of strong voices in neonatology, obstetric, public health, and nursing research is providing evidence that the consequences of *racism*, and not race per se, negatively affect health outcomes for Black women and their infants.[5] The United States ranks fifty-seventh in the world for infant mortality, and the United States ranks sixty-fifth among industrialized nations in terms of maternal death.[6] A large body of research focuses on the existence and persistence of health disparities in pregnancy outcomes related to infants, such as mortality, preterm birth, and breastfeeding rates. However, maternal outcomes have significantly worsened in the past twenty years, with increases in cesarean section births, early elective deliveries, severe complications, and death. Moreover, maternal complications are the fourth leading cause of infant death.[7] For most perinatal quality indicators, Black women and their infants experience worse outcomes than do white women and infants.[8] Most concerning is that pregnancy-related deaths occur among Black women at four to five times the rate among white women.

Ideas about racialized or "other" bodies that are "clinically" known but based on cultural beliefs have a long history in medicine. These ideas take hold as "facts," yet are not derived from scientific evidence.[9] Research by Kelly M. Hoffman and colleagues provides "evidence that false beliefs about biological differences between blacks and whites continue to shape the way we perceive and treat black people—they are associated with racial disparities in pain assessment and treatment recommendations."[10] While the relationship between pain and racial bias occurs in all medical specialties, scholars draw connections between the particularly pernicious and racist past of obstetrics and its connection to the persistent and serious racial disparities in maternal and neonatal outcomes. Historian Deirdre Cooper Owens examines a wide range of scientific literature and informal communications in which physicians created, disseminated, and justified false beliefs that Black enslaved women could withstand pain better than white "ladies."[11] Physicians such as nineteenth-century South Carolina surgeon J. Marion Sims performed countless surgeries on enslaved women to "advance" the practice of gynecology. In reality, these doctors were legitimizing baseless theories related to whiteness and blackness, men and women, and the inferiority of nonwhite races or non-U.S. nationalities. These ideas about racial inferiority continue to affect medical and reproductive care today. Many of these ideas are now also thought of as a "hidden curriculum" in which medical students learn acceptable ways to continue perpetuating false ideas about race.

Medical Science and the Production of Knowledge

To our knowledge, the only mention of the phrase "wimpy white boy" in medical journals is in an editorial called "WWBS: Fact or Fiction," published in 2014 by David Oelberg in the *Journal of Perinatology—Neonatology*. Oelberg defines wimpy white boy syndrome as "a neonatal white boy with adjusted gestational age of 35–40 weeks who is failing to achieve the developmental landmarks of weaning to an open crib and/or taking all of his oral feeds as expected" and clarifies that this is not an *ICD-10* coded diagnosis, meaning a diagnosis, symptom, or procedure recognized in the *International Classification of Diseases, Tenth Edition*, used by providers and hospitals to record and bill for services.[12] According to Oelberg, the phrase came into use in 2007 on lay websites, and he asserts that "there are no observational studies confirming the existence of [wimpy white boy syndrome]." He found the phrase potentially offensive but also thought that it might be valuable to investigate the phenomenon more. He clarified that in order to study this phenomenon, a study design should include standardized practices around feeding and weaning at all units for all babies, which is largely impossible due to variation between and within NICUs.[13]

The medical literature examining sex and/or race differences in neonatal morbidity or mortality varies in terms of what questions are asked and which gestational ages or weight categories are included, making it challenging to summarize the research overall. A smaller group of studies looks specifically at race and gender differences in lung disease morbidities, a diagnostic category in which males are considered largely disadvantaged. We found just one study whose results do not support the claim that there is a sex- and race-based disadvantage for white males.[14] When studies looked at sex and/or race for differences, the outcome of interest varied but typically included neonatal mortality. Two studies found a lower neonatal mortality risk for Black premature and low birthweight infants than for white premature and low birthweight infants and also found that this advantage for white babies continued into higher gestational age and birthweights.[15] Another study claimed a morbidity and mortality advantage for preterm females in general.[16]

In an often-cited 2006 article on the observation of frailty among white boys in the NICU, Steven B. Morse looked at one-year survival rates among extremely low birthweight infants (birthweights between 300 and 1,000 grams, or less than one to just over two pounds). Morse found that Black female infants had the greatest odds of survival and white male infants the worst across all weight ranges.[17] According to Morse, the order of decreasing survival rates at all gestational ages and weights was Black female, white female, Black male, and white male. These differences in survival were greater at lower gestational ages. Another study, by Ryan Loftin, found that between thirty-two and thirty-seven weeks gestational age, *Black infants had a lower frequency* of adverse neonatal outcomes than white infants but that after thirty-seven weeks, white infants had lower frequencies of adverse neonatal outcomes than Black infants.[18]

Greg R. Alexander found that Black infants had a lower risk of infant mortality if they were preterm and low birthweight compared to white and Hispanic infants.[19]

Racial and sex disparities in lung development are often cited as possible reasons for racial or sex disparities in outcomes in very low birthweight or preterm infants. This literature can be divided into two types of studies: those that focus on sex and those that focus on race or ethnicity. Courtney Townsel provided a review of research on sex disparities in preterm respiratory morbidity and mortality, finding that, overall, males had higher respiratory morbidity and mortality relative to females in both the very low birthweight and late preterm categories.[20] Additionally, we identified a body of research on racial disparities following the late 1980s introduction of surfactant, a steroid medication used to help with lung development for preterm infants, that supports this view. Aaron Hamvas found that surfactants' ability to improve mortality was more pronounced in white than Black very low birthweight (VLBW) neonates.[21] Similarly, in a 2000 study, Deepa Ranganathan found that from 1988 to 1991, upon the introduction of surfactant, there was an increased decline in neonatal mortality due to respiratory distress syndrome and deaths due to respiratory causes for non-Hispanic white VLBW infants weighing 750 to 1,250 g relative to African American infants.[22] In 2004, W. Parker Frisbie found that in the post-surfactant era, Black infants went from a survival advantage to a survival disadvantage relative to whites.[23] However, not all research on surfactant use monitors the historical impact of surfactant. Elizabeth Howell, who tested whether there were racial or ethnic disparities in the *administration* of surfactant when equally indicated, found a disadvantage for Black or African American infants, who did not receive equal standard of care.[24]

We identified only one study that explicitly challenged the idea of white male infant fragility in NICU outcomes. In 2002, five years before Oelberg claimed that WWBS emerged from lay websites, Jana Pressler and Joseph Hepworth addressed what they called a "common belief" among nurse caregivers about the disadvantage that white male infants experience by being "more medically fragile and at higher risk for morbidities than other preterm infants."[25] Stating that no evidence exists to support the belief of white male infant fragility, the authors noted that while gender and race differences have been found in other studies, these studies looked at outcomes after NICU care, not outcomes in the NICU. Pressler and Hepworth conducted their own newborn behavioral research focused on developmental goals, and they did not find empirical support for what they called the "Caucasian male infant hypothesis."

Neonatal Clinicians and Parents Talk about Wimpy White Boy Syndrome

Neonatal clinicians we spoke with were familiar with the wimpy white boy syndrome meme and introduced clinical observations and population data that demonstrate a female advantage over males in terms of mortality rates and other markers. However, most clinicians cautioned against using population data to predict an individual outcome, and many expressed discomfort with the term "wimpy." Clinical observations were cited as one source of data that lent truth to the wimpy white boy syndrome. One neonatologist asserted, "You definitely see it clinically. We definitely see that the boys are sometimes not as vigorous early on and you just see that clinically."

Some neonatologists tempered their statements about clinical observations of a disadvantage by focusing on generalities rather than particular types of morbidities or specific gestational ages. After we asked for those types of specifics, one physician responded, "It [wimpy white boy syndrome] doesn't have any one thing in particular, you know, the same things that we always get, like infections, or a brain bleed, or some other complication that you associate with prematurity, then you want to know who's hit the hardest, and who's probably going to bounce back. You know, these are all just generalizations, you can't really apply them to any specific baby."

We found that neonatal clinicians who responded to our request to tell us about wimpy white boy syndrome responded in two distinct ways. Some discounted sex and race as relevant markers in the care they provided to infants, while others argued for the utility of specific sex and race profiles associated with poor outcomes. As one clinician remarked, "The phrase in general, forget about your color of your skin. The girls, you know, are sometimes—can be a little more resilient, it seems, but whatever. I mean, none of it is useful." Several clinicians expressed discomfort with actually using the term in conversation with parents, because sex and race are not modifiable factors and thus do not drive care decisions or quality improvement. Said another clinician, "Actually, when I talk to parents, I try not to talk to them about nonmodifiable things. To say 'gee, if you were just a girl' or 'gee, Aren't you lucky that you're black', or something like that. We've heard it that way too. Yeah. That takes you down a rabbit hole that is probably not doing anybody any good."

Many neonatal clinicians used vague phrases when talking about wimpy white boy syndrome, such as, "some babies do better" or "worse" than others or may need more "support." A nurse clarified what they meant and went on to note that "across the board," it is health acuity, or severity, that matters: "When

I talk about them doing well . . . or the amount of support that they need, I think about medical support. . . . So, do they need a ventilator, do they need vasopressors or blood or . . . ? These are all things that nurses provide the care for. But that kind of medical support suggests higher morbidity factors that *go across the board*. It doesn't matter what the ethnicity, the higher acuity of the patient, the more worried we are about their outcomes."

Another clinician responded to our question about how neonatal outcomes vary by race or ethnicity and sex by taking it a step further, to say that there should be race and sex profiles but that these two factors should be considered alongside a whole list of relevant social and clinical factors, such as mother's health status, baby's clinical presentation, family socioeconomic status, social support, and lactation support, for example.[26] For this neonatologist, the race and sex of an infant seem to influence morbidities in ways that are not always taken into account. They saw this through the lens of quality improvement, in that NICUs are liable to, for example, over- or underestimate quality improvement success given that the race and sex risk profiles of their patient population are not taken into account. When we asked this neonatologist about whether wimpy white boy syndrome figures into how infants are treated, they told us,

> Well, I think it should, right, because when I do rounds and I hear about the pneumothorax [collapsed lung] in white babies. . . . It sort of evolved into my declaring that we really don't know how to provide good care to the white male infant and . . . if a pneumothorax can happen, we will let it happen. So I still believe that there is a risk reduction approach that maybe we're not careful enough or we're doing something wrong. But I'm usually holding my team to that standard of, you know, [white boys] is the highest risk group [for pneumothorax]. So we have to be even more judicious in doing better since we know that these kids are at risk. I think my language seeks to imply that if you're a high risk group and I'm aware of that, then I should be able to have targeted risk reduction strategies for you—maybe I should be a bit more proactive . . . maybe I should get that x-ray sooner.

This neonatologist saw gender/race risk profiles as just two dimensions to include in neonatal risk profiles and was hesitant to elevate WWBS above other types. "Well, you know," they said, "disparities in the African American community are the most severe, whether it's sudden infant death or it's mortality rate at prematurity or infant mortality, period. . . . So I don't want to leave out the black community and make this a white boy issue because every race and every group has its own risk profile."

Like clinicians, parents (mostly mothers) who took part in discussion boards on premature birth largely offered explanations of wimpy white boy syndrome that affirmed its empirical basis, as they understood it. Whereas clinicians referred to their clinical experiences and observations, parents shared their lived experiences. In one baby forum discussion, the original poster asked whether anyone had previously heard about wimpy white boy syndrome, and 83 percent of the thirty-seven who answered said they knew about it before reading the post. As they shared their experiences, some parents indicated who told them about wimpy white boy syndrome. As one parent noted, "My oldest was a preemie and in the NICU for ten days. I can't remember if any of the nurses used this term but I was told that male Caucasian babies do seem to struggle the most." Another parent noted that her boy was premature and admitted to the NICU, where, she said, "The doctor joked had he been a girl, he probably wouldn't have spent any time there. I was all confused and he explained . . . Black girls are the strongest and white boys are wimps."

Several parents responded to the potential fear or concern that might arise when hearing that one's infant is disadvantaged by sex and race by telling a counternarrative about their experience, or by drawing on statistical understandings, to say that overall data are not predictive for individuals over the long term. The mother of one wimpy white boy noted, "He hit all his milestones late and had me very concerned but he finally caught up on everything around 20 months. But major milestones like rolling, sitting up, crawling, cruising, and walking were months behind his peers." Other parents offered stories about infants other than their own, comparing the outcomes of black and white infants: "My guys were 30 weekers. One was in the hospital for 5 weeks the other was in for 8 weeks. At the same time, there was a set of 24 weeker African American identical twin girls, that were about the same gestational age as my boys. They went home before they even hit 4 lb! I got to be buddies with their dad, and those amazing little girls were MUCH stronger than my guys."

When parents shared "exceptions to the rule," they often offered assurances that not all white male infants experience WWBS and that white males do have good outcomes nevertheless. One parent posted about her white male twins not being wimpy: "I was very surprised. They were only in the NICU for 11 and 13 days, which is pretty good for their gestational age (33w2d)." Parents of boy/girl twins provided exception stories, such as "statistically speaking, this is true . . . but it was the complete opposite for our b/g twins in the NICU. So you never know, each baby is so different. Don't let the statistic discourage you!"

Not Useful for Prognosis or Quality Improvement—and Potentially Harmful

All neonatologists were critical of the phrase and told us that they do not use the term. As one said, "When I hear people say those sorts of things, it makes me wince." One of the posters in the parent discussion was herself a neonatal clinician and noted, "It's unfortunately a true statistic. NICU nurse here. I've never said it in front of a parent and I never will. I've never heard the doctors say it in that way to a parent either."

Other neonatologists noted the detrimental effect of labeling infants in this way and pointed out that labeling is not good practice in most parenting situations. Reinforcing ideas that the infant is weak may affect parenting in the NICU and after discharge to home. One neonatologist whose research focuses on family psychological support noted the connection between strong parent-infant bonds and long-term outcomes for infants. Rather than use a term that connotes weakness, they advised, "You know, helping parents reframe as the 'baby is strong' and capable and things like that, can actually help them bond to their kids."

Clinicians acknowledged the "politically incorrect" nature of wimpy white boy syndrome, but parents' posts demonstrate how they hear and react to their infant described in those terms. The term "wimpy" was problematic for one parent, who noted that "I got a white little boy and he's definitely not weak. He's pulled major chunks of my hair out. That's a stupid name for a syndrome. If a nurse had said that about my little one I would've been pretty irritated." Several parents expanded on the idea that the name is "stupid," or "unhelpful"; as one mother noted, "I'm sure babies of other races and genders have been 'wimpy' as well. Why even make up an offensive term just because a certain type of baby gets it more often?" Some parents responded with even stronger emotions: "I had a nurse say this to me when I almost had my son at 24 weeks. I wanted to punch her cause I was already scared to death of him dying. I told the charge nurse to please take note I never want her around me again." Another noted that clinicians sometimes "don't think before they say things that might scare a new mom!!!"

A Useless, Political Hot Potato

In the larger scheme of neonatal outcomes, neonatologists downplayed wimpy white boy syndrome as something meriting further study, as compared to research or quality improvement projects focused on specifics, such as lung complications, central line infections, and other serious clinical scenarios. "It's interesting to have this discussion, but because we're having this discussion, it is brought to the forefront. I think that when you're on the front lines and doing the actual work, it's not a concept that percolates into your top ten or whatever, you know," one clinician said. A neonatologist noted that it was difficult to imagine how addressing WWBS would affect neonatal outcomes from a quality improvement perspective, when there are more opportunities for NICUs to improve care with respect to issues such as breastmilk feeding rates and infection rates. They said, "If you're poking around looking for differences, but don't have an action or some set of action plan associated package to make things better, it gets you pretty far upstream and there's such a world of things where there are tool kits and we've just got to get people to use them." In other words, addressing "upstream" issues such as sex and race requires examining cultural and social determinants of health, which, while important, did not seem a priority to this clinician when compared with implementing quality initiatives that could have more immediate impact.

A few clinicians warned us about possible negative consequences that might ensue if WWBS became a primary focus of research. "It'll be interesting how this particular work gets perceived when you turn it over to the general populace," one said, reflecting concerns that this research could be interpreted in ways that put neonatology in a bad light. As one neonatologist said, "I think [your research question] is interesting; I'm not sure I've ever seen this put down on paper. I don't think that's an accident." Others were concerned about how findings from this study might be skewed if it attracted media attention: "There are potential pitfalls in the way it can be presented and interpreted. When you talk about race in this country, it's never an easy discussion. When you talk about some kind of racial superiority I think you're going to get a lot of pushback. You're going to get strong emotional responses that aren't based on anything other than emotion." One parent foreshadowed this in her comment: "I don't find wimpy white boy syndrome offensive, but I know that if there was a NICU term called 'wimpy black boy' or something along those lines then all hell would break loose."

Much of the concern about negative media attention reflects the fact that many white people in health care fields have challenges talking about race. Our respondents discussed sex differences among neonates without problems, but some were openly uncomfortable speaking about race, racism, or race relations directly. One neonatologist told us that they do not talk about race, in part because the data are not conclusive but also because race is hard to talk about: "I found myself over the years in struggling a bit with how to approach race because it is such, you know, such a socially difficult thing to deal with."

In addition to the problematics of race as a topic in health care discussions generally, all of the neonatal clinicians we spoke with acknowledged that the phrase "wimpy white boy" is passé and not politically correct or clinically useful. Most said they do not hear the term on a regular basis in clinical practice. This may be due to the patient mix of the NICUs where they work, whether one looks at race or socioeconomic factors. Some of the clinicians we spoke with worked with very few Black patients. All of the neonatal clinicians said they thought that wimpy white boy syndrome does not affect quality of care in NICUs where they work, saying things such as, "We treat everyone the same," or "I don't think about gender." Yet in the same breath, they raised the issue of socioeconomic status, another salient factor in quality of care disparities.

Parents with critical views took issue not just with the term "wimpy" but also its connotations about racial identity or other stigmatized terms that are no longer appropriate in professional discourses. "I think the first few weeks postpartum are an especially vulnerable time for women and I would hate to think of someone who might already be struggling to hear these words. It brings to mind the word retarded," one parent noted. Acknowledging the current racial climate, another parent remarked, "I had never heard of that syndrome; it just sounds demeaning. I could only imagine if there were a 'wimpy black kid' or 'limpy [sic] Latin kid' syndrome. I'm sure 'White America' would be blamed for the reference. Oh . . . the pandemonium that would unleash due to the negative stigma associated with this 'medical' terminology." One parent poster suggested such terms might have a reach beyond health care: "Those nurses who use this term in front of patients aren't helping with the racial tension in this country!"

Discussions about whether wimpy white boy syndrome was racist often included posts from parents who provided justifications for its underlying intention and use in a clinical context. One said, "It's a true statement even if the words are not politically correct. No offense taken here. It is what it is." Some also redefined what "wimpy" meant in the NICU setting, where, they believed, the usual social norms do not apply: "If I called someone a 'wimp' it would be meant as an insult—or at least emasculating. But in THIS medical context, I would understand that term to suggest 'an underdog.' And don't we all root for the underdog?"

To clinicians, wimpy white boy syndrome also raises the possibility of setting up expectations that white boys are the weakest and need the most support, which may affect clinical decisions. Reflected one clinician, "Well, if you have a strong feeling that girls do better than boys and if a girl's going through a rough patch, you may push yourself harder in some way to make that child better—or be less willing to let go if things are going terribly because girls shouldn't die, you know." We wondered whether the opposite might happen, that due to beliefs about wimpy white boy syndrome, premature or low birth-weight Black girls might get less clinical attention. When we raised this issue, one neonatologist reflected,

> In our society, it's hardest for black women, for black females . . . : I think that's not new, special or different. And I think in order to get to this point, there had to be something inherent in them (black females) for sur-vivability because, like, the odds were not in their favor. You know, in the *Hunger Games,* they say "May the odds ever be in your favor." The odds were not in their favor. I think the weakness probably gets weeded out to some degree, because it doesn't make it. I think you're allowed [to] be kind of wimpy or weak if you have a lot of support around you.

Importantly, not all clinicians we spoke to saw wimpy white boy syndrome as a cause for additional treatment or concern for white male infants. Rather, some theorized that some neonatal clinicians might respond with undertreat-ment or reduced concern by framing it as a typical but ultimately benign issue, telling worried parents, "It is *just* a wimpy white boy. Don't worry."

Problematic Cultural Resonance

Beyond that of a "political hot potato," we are concerned about the problem-atic way that the concept of WWBS correlates with Black infant girls described as "stronger" due to evolutionary factors or social determinants, and that white infant boys described as "allowed to be wimpy or weak" because they are in a supportive environment. In the current U.S. culture, the idea that white boys are in need of greater support flies in the face of very real economic and social indicators that place white males at the top. Furthermore, framing premature Black infant girls as "strong" plays into stereotypes that white culture has used when describing Black women. Scholars have challenged the notion of the "strong Black woman" and or a Black "superwoman schema" unpacking its his-torical and cultural resonance.[27] In a study that connects historical notions of Black womanhood and the influence of Black culture on Black women's ideals about body image, Beauboeuf-Lafontant found that these "ideals" not only affect women's health outcomes, most particularly mental illness and eating disorders, but also falsely ascribe emotional and spiritual strength to Black women. When Black women are expected to embody emotional toughness and a survivor men-tality, and when this expectation is also placed on the premature Black female infant, the health consequences can be grave. Black women are caught in a double bind, as within Black culture, they are expected to typify the selfless, forever giving, passive nurturer, mother figure who never gives anything in return, while in the NICU, as premature babies, they were expected to be tough, scrappy survivors.[28]

Conclusion

Our investigation into wimpy white boy syndrome revealed that its clinical parameters are not well established, and the research cited in support of it looks primarily at broad neonatal outcomes, such as severe morbidity or mortality. In the absence of data to demonstrate whether and how infant sex and race may impact quality of care, we raise concerns about using memes such as wimpy white boy syndrome in clinical discussions, or even pursuing the question further as a research topic.

Even if there is quality research demonstrating that white boys are diagnosed with respiratory illnesses due to differences in lung development, extending metaphoric ideas about strength and weakness is not useful information for parents, and as our data show, may be viewed as offensive or racist. Although quality of care of babies in the NICU varies by infant race, nearly all clinicians volunteered their opinions that the baby sex does not affect the care their units provide. Neonatal clinicians stressed that the baby's clinical status determines treatment needs, yet it is difficult to imagine that ideas about the relative 'strength' or 'weakness' of a baby based on race do not have some impact on clinical behavior.

Wimpy white boy syndrome centers white boys while contrasting them most explicitly with black girls. The concept largely overlooks white girls and black boys, however, and furthermore, it reduces racial groupings to black and white, obscuring other possible differences in quality of care for Asian and Hispanic infants, for example. Race in America has always prioritized black-white relationships. Meanwhile, the question remains: is the wimpy white boy syndrome an empirical phenomenon? The question may never be adequately addressed in research. For us, the more important question is how to identify the structures and processes that underlie persistent, significant disparities in NICU outcomes and quality of care in order to ensure that all babies, regardless of sex or race, are cared for in the best possible way.

Notes

1. We identified potential neonatal clinicians through existing professional networks. We purposely selected for diverse identities, including men, women, white, Black, and U.S.- and foreign-born and trained clinicians, and those in different regions. All clinicians who were invited to participate agreed to do so, and we conducted

interviews by telephone or videoconference in the spring and summer of 2019. Because we assured clinicians anonymity and confidentiality, and because this is a small professional network, we do not note their names, roles, or individual characteristics when quoting them.

2. Krista Sigurdson et al., "Racial/Ethnic Disparities in Neonatal Intensive Care: A Systematic Review," *Pediatrics* 144, no. 2 (2019).

3. Wanda D. Barfield, S. Cox, and Z. T. Henderson, "Disparities in Neonatal Intensive Care: Context Matters," *Pediatrics* 144, no. 2 (2019).

4. BabyCenter.com, https://community.babycenter.com/post/a53573026/wimpy_white _boy_syndrome; The Bump https://forums.thebump.com/discussion/1144362/quot -wimpy-white-boys-quot-more-nicu-time.

5. Monica R. McLemore, "To Prevent Women from Dying in Childbirth, First Stop Blaming Them," *Scientific American*, May 1, 2019; Joia Crear-Perry, "Race Isn't a Risk Factor in Maternal Health. Racism Is," *Rewire.News*, April 11, 2018; Monica R. McLemore et al., "Health Care Experiences of Pregnant, Birthing and Postnatal Women of Color at Risk for Preterm Birth," *Social Science & Medicine* 201 (2018).

6. Centers for Disease Control and Prevention, "Reproductive Health, Pregnancy Mortality Surveillance System Webpage," https://www.cdc.gov/reproductivehealth/matern alinfanthealth/pregnancy-mortality-surveillance-system.htm.

7. Hsiang-Ching Kung et al., "Deaths: Preliminary Data for 2005" *Health E-Stats* (2007).

8. E. E. Petersen, N. L. Davis, D. Goodman, S. Cox, C. Syverson, K. Seed, C. Shapiro-Mendoza, W. M. Callaghan, and W. Barfield, "Racial/Ethnic Disparities in Pregnancy-Related Deaths—United States, 2007–2016," *MMWR Morbidity and Mortality Weekly Report* 68, no. 35 (2019): 762–65.

9. Harriet A. Washington, *Medical Apartheid: The Dark History of Medical Experimentation on Black Americans from Colonial Times to the Present* (New York: Doubleday, 2006).

10. Kelly M. Hoffman et al., "Racial Bias in Pain Assessment and Treatment Recommendations, and False Beliefs About Biological Differences between Blacks and Whites," *Proceedings of the National Academy of Sciences U S A* 113, no. 16 (2016).

11. Deirdre Cooper Owens, *Medical Bondage: Race, Gender, and the Origins of American Gynecology* (Athens: University of Georgia Press, 2017).

12. David G. Oelberg, "WWBS: Fact or Fiction?" *Neonatal Intensive Care* 27, no. 2 (2014).

13. Jochen Profit et al., "Racial/Ethnic Disparity in NICU Quality of Care Delivery," *Pediatrics* 140, no. 3 (2017).

14. Jana L. Pressler and Joseph T. Hepworth, "A Quantitative Use of the NIDCAP® Tool: The Effect of Gender and Race on Very Preterm Neonates' Behavior," *Clinical Nursing Research* 11, no. 1 (2002).

15. William M. Sappenfield et al., "Differences in Neonatal and Postneonatal Mortality by Race, Birth Weight, and Gestational Age," *Public Health Report* 102, no. 2 (1987); Greg R. Alexander et al., "US Birth Weight/Gestational Age-Specific Neonatal Mortality: 1995–1997 Rates for Whites, Hispanics, and Blacks," *Pediatrics* 111, no. 1 (2003).

16. David K. Stevenson et al., "Sex Differences in Outcomes of Very Low Birthweight Infants: The Newborn Male Disadvantage," *Archives of Disease in Childhood—Fetal and Neonatal Edition* 83, no. 3 (2000).

17. Steven B. Morse et al., "Racial and Gender Differences in the Viability of Extremely Low Birth Weight Infants: A Population-Based Study," *Pediatrics* 117, no. 1 (2006).

18. Ryan Loftin et al., "Racial Differences in Gestational Age-Specific Neonatal Morbidity: Further Evidence for Different Gestational Lengths," *American Journal of Obstetrics and Gynecology* 206, no. 3 (2012).

19. Alexander et al., "US Birth Weight/Gestational Age-Specific Neonatal Mortality."

20. Courtney Denise Townsel et al., "Gender Differences in Respiratory Morbidity and Mortality of Preterm Neonates," *Frontiers in Pediatrics* 5 (2017).

21. Aaron Hamvas et al., "The Influence of the Wider Use of Surfactant Therapy on Neonatal Mortality among Blacks and Whites," *New England Journal of Medicine* 334, no. 25 (1996).

22. Deepa Ranganathan et al., "Racial Differences in Respiratory-Related Neonatal Mortality among Very Low Birth Weight Infants," *Journal of Pediatrics* 136, no. 4 (2000).

23. W. Parker Frisbie et al., "The Increasing Racial Disparity in Infant Mortality: Respiratory Distress Syndrome and Other Causes," *Demography* 41, no. 4 (2004).

24. Elizabeth A. Howell et al., "Surfactant Use for Premature Infants with Respiratory Distress Syndrome in Three New York City Hospitals: Discordance of Practice from a Community Clinician Consensus Standard," *Journal of Perinatology* 30, no. 9 (2010).

25. Pressler and Hepworth, "A Quantitative Use of the NIDCAP® Tool."

26. In the early 2000s, the NICHD Neonatal Research Network (NRN) developed an algorithm that helps guide clinicians as they counsel parents on outcomes associated with preterm birth. Using Extremely Preterm Birth Outcome Data, the tool asks for fields such as gestational age, birthweight, sex, single or multiple birth, and whether antenatal corticosteroids were administered within seven days of the birth. Interestingly, the tool does not ask for race/ethnicity. The website stresses that "these data are not intended to predict individual infant outcomes" but does suggest that sex data are meaningful for neonatologists who use this tool. U.S. Department of Health and Human Services, National Institutes of Health, "NICHD Neonatal Research Network (Nrn): Extremely Preterm Birth Outcome Data," https://www1.nichd.nih.gov /epbo-calculator/Pages/epbo_case.aspx.

27. Amani M. Allen, Yijie Wang, David H. Chae, Melisa M. Price, Wizdom Powell, Teneka C. Steed, Angela Rose Black, et al. "Racial Discrimination, the Superwoman Schema, and Allostatic Load: Exploring an Integrative Stress-Coping Model among African American Women," *Annals of the New York Academy of Sciences* 1457, no. 1 (2019): 104–27.

28. Tamara Beauboeuf-Lafontant, "You Have to Show Strength: An Exploration of Gender, Race, and Depression," *Gender & Society* 21, no. 1 (2007).

Part 2

Body Politic

Chapter 7

Masculinity and the Case for a Childhood Vaccine

Elena Conis

When an outbreak causing swollen jaws and testicles of "a frightful enormous magnitude" spread among the soldiers under his care in 1761, British physician Robert Hamilton searched "in vain" for clinical histories and cures. Finding little, and eventually "reduced to the utmost danger" by the affliction himself, Hamilton summarized his observations for "future observers." He painted a picture of an apparently new fever that affected children only mildly but caused debilitation and disorder when it erupted among men; the "common people of England," he noted, called it mumps.[1] From the publication of his observations in 1790 to the U.S. licensure of the modern mumps vaccine in 1967, Hamilton was often granted credit for documenting and describing the disease. In the era of mumps vaccination, however, he was gradually forgotten; in the United States in particular, the details of mumps' clinical history became subordinated to the push to encourage the vaccination of children against the disease in the 1970s. But in forgetting Hamilton, American medicine and public health also forgot a long history of disagreement over the very nature of mumps. These disagreements concerned who mumps most threatened and whose cases ought therefore to be prevented—and they reveal that sex and gender mattered significantly in nearly two centuries of clinical and popular assessments of mumps.

This essay takes Hamilton's account as a starting point for analyzing mumps' prevaccine history in the West, with a focus on the United States, to show how gender rendered mumps medically, politically, and economically insignificant, or invisible, in some patients and far more significant in others. From Hamilton's time to the early years of mumps vaccination in the United States, mumps was considered a problem that primarily concerned adolescent boys and adult

men, and men's experiences with the disease in military contexts in particular
drove the development of mumps vaccines—for men. By the 1970s, however,
the most effective of those vaccines would come to be a routine part of pediatric care, administered to all American children, regardless of sex. This essay
argues that the timing of that vaccine's development and approval helped transform mumps itself from a serious disease of men to a serious disease of all
children. The long history of mumps leading up to the development of its first
effective vaccine also shows how the sociocultural politics of gender quietly
shaped the use of a childhood vaccine adopted well before the development of
childhood vaccines against sexually transmitted infections, such as hepatitis B
virus and human papillomavirus (HPV), whose histories as gendered objects
have already been explored.[2]

Hamilton's 1790 report described mumps as a disease "generally confined to
young men, from the age of puberty upwards to thirty years"; he claimed he
never saw a case in "any of the female sex above ten years old." The disease's
painful testicular "tumors" were its most "dreadful symptoms," and he described
some of the worst cases he had seen, including those that ended in permanently
diminished testicles and death.[3] Looking back to Hippocrates for etiological
explanation, Hamilton found description of an ancient epidemic that caused
"swelling about the ears" and occasional pain and inflammation in one or both
testicles but "seldom attacked women." The chief victims were children and
adults—namely, men—who exercised in the gymnasium. Hamilton proposed a
miasmatic explanation of the mumps, seeing his soldiers, like Hippocrates' subjects, as susceptible because they were "out early and late in the low damp
grounds . . . to learn their manual exercise."[4] In Hamilton's assessment, gendered
patterns of activity rendered men vulnerable to the disease; he noted that his
own military men rarely seemed to pass the disease to their wives and children,
protected by sex or age from the miasmatic exposures of war.

Mumps, new to Hamilton, would come of age in the century of industrialization, growth, and medical professionalization that followed, by the end of
which hundreds of reports in Western medical journals described its features,
epidemiology, and complications. Most were case reports offering descriptions
of mumps' rare complications: enlarged or suppurating glands, deafness, testicular atrophy, and insanity. A significant number described epidemics striking burgeoning cities and towns and growing institutions of learning, production, and
confinement, sites where primarily men congregated. In the bulk of nineteenth-
century medical literature—and news reports—covering mumps, mumps was of
more interest as a disease of men than a disease of women or children.

Medical writers who *did* discuss children's mumps in the nineteenth century described it, as Hamilton did, as "mild" and "benign": it was not fatal in its "uncomplicated" form, did not spread as far and wide as smallpox, and did not stop children from "getting out of bed" or "engaging in their usual occupations and games."[5] It seemed to be common among children who spent time crowded in schools and nurseries; because it struck "but once during life," it appeared more often among children than adults. Mumps was so common among children by midcentury that one newspaper suggested someone organize a place for parents to have their children infected at a convenient time, so they could "be disposed of [it] for life."[6] In fact, children's mumps were considered so harmless they even constituted a source of amusement, with papers offering funny stories of swollen-faced girls and boys.[7] If children's cases were comical, women's were mysterious, in part because they seemed so rare. Early nineteenth-century medical journals offered conflicting accounts of the female body parts affected by mumps: breasts, ovaries, or labia. Where the disease did seem to inflame such organs, physicians reported no lasting effects. Some dismissed the contested complications as myths modern physicians should abandon as relics of the "authority of the traditional woman."[8] Others speculated that female physiology or modesty kept mumps' true effects on the female body undetectable.[9] Newspaper writers mentioned women's mumps only when it disrupted their roles as caregivers or objects of beauty or entertainment. So it went with Princess Victoria's mumps, which reportedly so incensed Queen Victoria that she banned from Windsor Castle the young child who brought it into the household. Mumps was, after all, an "unbecoming complaint" for a princess, an American reporter noted.[10]

Neither medical nor popular observers called mumps "unbecoming" among men. And while mumps in women stayed confined to individuals or households, men contracted mumps in congregations. The regiments with hundreds or thousands of cases in the U.S. Civil War made this clear.[11] Army camp illnesses were so common—disease killed twice as many soldiers as battle did—that mumps attracted little special attention among them, notable mostly for the debilitating pain its testicular complication caused.[12] Its prevalence also complicated debate over its contagious nature. The wartime spread of disease lent credence to the idea of contagion generally, although with respect to mumps, some held to the theory that hard army biscuits required bursts of "masticatory strength" that left the body sapped of energy and prone to disease. The same theory explained mumps' predilection for men, thanks to what one physician called "the increased excitability of the sexual organs in . . . men pent up or confined anywhere."[13] With the economic shifts that followed the war, young middle-class men rotated between home, college, boardinghouse, and other institutions, where they encountered other men in close confines that continued to foster mumps' spread.[14] As germ theory gained further credence in the century's final decades, doctors and bacteriologists began attempts to isolate a suspected "form of bacillus," relying on epidemics among students, quartered soldiers, and other institutionalized men.[15] The idea of mumps as a serious contagious disease thus took root in contexts that reified it as a particular threat to men.

Meanwhile, the pattern of representing mumps as a laughing matter among children and women persisted, even as evidence of more serious mumps sequelae accrued, and even as young women moved into spaces dominated by men, especially universities, where mumps affected both sexes.[16] By the late nineteenth century, the medical literature was peppered with cases of mumps complications ranging from pupil dilation and sensitivity to light to severe head pain, delirium, aphasia, sensory delusions, and even insanity.[17] But in a by-then entrenched pattern, the most dramatic of these complications were reported as if confined to men.[18] At a time when, as Mark S. Micale has argued, "the highly demarcated world of gender extensively shaped the medical discourse of the day," mumps filled a void left by the Victorian-era suppression of the idea of nervousness or hysteria in men, simultaneously fitting into the narratives of "passionate manhood" that defined the time.[19] Mumps-induced insanity in males was so accepted by the end of the century that it morphed into a medically and socially accepted explanation for a range of extreme behaviors, including dramatic and gruesome suicides in "prominent" men.[20] When a twenty-three-year-old Harvard student stabbed himself sixty-four times with a penknife, his father, president of New York's Broadway Underground Railroad, said his son had been driven mad by mumps.[21] Hysteria-like behaviors forced men out of the public sphere of power and productivity, but if the wandering womb explained mental aberrations in women, the unruly testicle could explain the same behaviors in men, its contagious nature a convenient exoneration from personal blame.

Micale's argument about the nineteenth-century submersion of male hysteria is supported by the condition's faint imprint in the medical literature. Mumps-induced insanity is similarly lightly imprinted, but the same seemed to be true of mumps generally in the late 1800s. To those who were intrigued by the disease, especially its unique manifestation in men, it was an overlooked malady. Writing of his town's bout with mumps-induced "derangement," a Nebraska physician found it odd that although mumps was "one of our most widely extended and frequently recurring epidemics," medical literature made little mention of it. A popular 3,000-page medical textbook devoted just one page to mumps; an 800-page textbook on the disease of children devoted only two.[22] A pair of physicians from New Jersey and Philadelphia found a similar pattern in bacteriology texts. The idea that mumps was caused by a "microbe" was firmly accepted by the very end of the century, but they found that "the text-books almost without exception ignore it entirely."[23]

In 1898, French mumps expert Jules Comby reviewed the medical litera-ture on mumps for the American medical text *Twentieth Century Practice*. He described it as a contagious infection that caused orchitis, or testicular swell-ing, in men and posed less clear consequences for women; was relatively rare and mild in children; and, if anything, was worse in boys, thanks to scarce cases of orchitis, than it ever seemed in girls. But he was skeptical of a sex difference. He noted that women had received far less attention than men as victims of the disease and that the "impression" that mumps struck boys more than girls "has been based on the statements of those who have studied epidemics in boys' schools and colleges." "If we leave aside statistics so gleaned," he wrote, "we shall see that this is an error." In a Geneva epidemic, males and females were affected in even proportions; in a Normandy epidemic, only women and children were struck. "Thus we see," he concluded, "that sex has no part in the etiology of mumps."[24]

At the end of a century in which, as Micale has put it, "medical science and practice were aggressively pressed into the service of discovering and main-taining a regime of difference between the sexes," Comby cast aside the idea of a sex difference with regards to mumps etiology.[25] But he retained a gendered understanding of mumps severity nonetheless, based entirely on the singular mumps complication to have become an "object of special study": orchitis. Although rare, orchitis could result in testicular atrophy, and atrophy could lead to "loss of virility, sterility, and an effeminacy of the constitution, as shown by the eunuch voice, enlargement of the breasts." He called these "the black spot in mumps in the adult," a conclusion that spoke directly to the centrality of the male body in late nineteenth-century conceptions of manhood.[26] Sex, for Comby, may have played no role in mumps' etiology, but its unique relationship with the still-elusive microbe posed a specific threat to masculinity.

Comby cautioned twentieth-century practitioners about mumps orchitis: "It is in the army especially that it is to be feared."[27] Mumps' spread in World War I proved him right. "Mumps again have appeared in the trenches," journalists reported from Berlin as World War I began.[28] A battalion commander in France said he had sent more men to the hospital for mumps than for enemy fire.[29] A year into the war, an American medical writer reported that the disease "ranked fifth among the causes of disability" in the U.S. Army."[30] The Civil War had confirmed mumps as a threat to armies of men; World War I now presented an urgent opportunity to study it as such.[31] Descriptive epidemiology revealed the first significant findings: military rates in war years far exceeded outbreaks in "child populations," and among troops, rural ones suffered most while urban men were generally protected.[32] Medical major Charles Sinclair calculated that the army saw more than 230,000 cases, each prompting an average of seventeen days of service lost, for a total of 4 million service days lost in the war.[33] Mumps, he concluded, "is a serious military disease by reason of its sick wastage."[34] Such wastage was not simply a matter of security but economy. A single epidemic affecting more than 21,000 men reportedly cost the U.S. Army more than $1 million in 1917. Mumps-affected men threatened to carry a postwar cost, too. A new federal agency was tasked with preventing the enormous financial outlays associated with veterans' disability that had followed the Civil War, and it embraced Progressive-era gender roles as it encouraged disabled soldiers returning from World War I to "marry, have children, and become breadwinners."[35] But what man with atrophied testicles could assume such a role?

With the war's end, as fatherhood became a growing subject of popular attention in the United States, so did mumps orchitis, previously taboo outside medical discourse.[36] Consistently, the complication was represented as a threat to fatherhood. Mumps had a "strong tendency toward involvement of the sexual glands," a complication that could "produce sterility," wrote popular medical writer Frank McCoy. Nervous young men, eager to experience the sense of masculine usefulness associated with interwar fathering, asked doctors if earlier mumps had left them sterile.[37] "If it were true that all cases of mumps develop into sterility, the human race would be but a fragment in numbers of what it is today," offered columnist Philip Lovell.[38] Lovell took the opportunity to call for the "average punster" to stop making fun of mumps, because it was "a tragedy to see a child with an atrophied testicle, compelled to go through life with his procreative functions either partly impaired on sometimes entirely destroyed."[39] Lovell projected the testicular complication and risk of sterility onto the male child, a conflation that would become more common as the twentieth century progressed, even as orchitis remained rare among the young and the risk of ensuing sterility remained unknown.

As mumps orchitis moved into public view in the 1920s and 1930s, doctors disputed how to characterize the disease: based on its benignity in children or its threat to reproductive organs in men. A series of *Washington Post* columns by two physicians captured the debate. To Irving Cutter, mumps was a "minor malady."[40] Logan Clendening, however, argued that "mumps is dangerous!" and "should be treated with great respect." He noted that George Washington had once said so and that "this might have been the reason Gen. Washington had no children."[41] Cutter disagreed; mumps "need not be serious," he wrote, noting that sterility occurred only "infrequently," even among those with severe testicular swelling.[42] Infrequent or not, "the complications make it important," Clendening rebuked, and mumps' return in times of war was guaranteed. But it was not a time of war, so he directed his opinions to the parents of children, namely sons: "As a word of advice to parents, do not regard mumps as trivial or a joke, and keep the child in bed for several days."[43] It was the best way to prevent testicular swelling, he urged.

Cutter and Clendening's mid-1930s debate followed an eventful decade for mumps. An outbreak in the isolated Faroe Islands had provided a unique opportunity to understand its effects among civilians. Boys and girls fell ill in equal numbers, but far more women than men fell sick. The physician who studied the epidemic thought males may have been protected by subclinical infections they acquired while off the islands for school and military service, picking up Comby's argument about gender roles. In the meantime, scientific disagreement over mumps' microbial agent came to a close as pathologists isolated the virus from university students and used it to infect seventeen children in a Tennessee town.[44] Mumps' dependable presence in young men and reputation as benign in young children justified the experimental methods, which, the researchers concluded, suggested a pathway toward possible "prophylaxis."[45] But with World War I a memory, there was little push for prophylaxis at the time. In popular and medical discourse, mumps remained "mild." "As a rule," wrote physician W. A. Evans, "parents do not dread it."[46]

War would once again change the conversation. A year after the United States entered World War II, army officials remarked that mumps incidence was low. "This is not surprising," wrote two Army Medical Corps majors, "when one considers the tremendous increase in travel during the past twenty-five years and the resultant decrease in isolation in rural areas."[47] On the whole, recruits seemed healthier than those who had served in World War I; less than 3 percent of soldiers were "noneffective" due to causes other than battle injuries.[48] In part, this was because army officials were more cautious, as approaches to mumps reveal: a single case or two now triggered quarantine for an entire battalion.[49] Still, the disease incapacitated thousands in camps across the country, and one officer noted that "almost every army post has had a certain number of cases."[50] Mumps may have been largely confined to children in peace, wrote pediatrician Joseph Stokes, but war was once again leading to "aggregation of susceptible" men. Mumps, along with measles, he argued, thus deserved to be a "major program" of the Army Epidemiological Board.[51]

This time around, army doctors and medics, some led by Stokes, made more deeply detailed studies of mumps in troops. In a Camp McCoy, Wisconsin, epidemic, orchitis occurred in 36 percent of cases, and meningoencephalitis occurred in 4 percent, a rate "very much more frequent than generally supposed."[52] British Army physicians observed that it did not even appear necessary for a man to have parotitis (swollen salivary glands) or orchitis for his mumps infection to lead to "meningeal symptoms."[53] The signs included disorientation, drowsiness, and twitching facial muscles; a diagnosis of "mental confusion" now began to supplant the mumps-induced "derangement" recorded the century before. More important, argued two physicians, since parotitis was not a defining aspect of the disease, it should be considered a complication, just as orchitis and encephalitis were.[54] The suggestion began to redefine mumps as a disease known for an array of complications, orchitis prominent among them. And now that the viral cause was known, a vaccine, of course, would prevent mumps from causing such complications in training camps, argued virologist Karl Habel, who was developing one at the National Institutes of Health.[55]

The first mumps vaccine was conceived as a prophylaxis for armies of men, but the scale of World War II amplified mumps as a matter of public health for men back home, too. Cases spiked in states like California, where it broke out among military personnel and defense workers recruited from rural areas.[56] Mumps ran rampant through factories and workcamps staffed with "shiploads" of men recruited from the West Indies to meet wartime labor needs.[57] Among the thousands of men from Barbados housed in nine agricultural workcamps bordering Lake Okeechobee, Florida, so many fell ill that one whole camp was designated a mumps infirmary. The unaffected men in such workcamps provided Habel and colleagues accessible, all-male populations in which to test their experimental vaccine. Their tests showed that the vaccine did not offer a high rate of protection, but among the vaccinated men who got mumps, the cases were milder and orchitis was half as common as it was among unvaccinated men who got sick.[58]

But with war's end, mumps vaccine proponents struggled to position the infection as "a disease to be regarded seriously" in soldiers *and* children.[59] At the first American Academy of Pediatrics (AAP) meeting after the war, a Harvard biologist who had spent the war studying mumps suggested diagnostic tests to separate susceptibles from the immune so that the vaccine could be used selectively in "children's institutions" and "Army camps" alike.[60] A different attitude prevailed at an AAP meeting a few years later. Three mumps vaccines were then in trials, but virologists Gertrude and Werner Henle warned that they "should never be employed indiscriminately."[61] A new combined vaccine against diphtheria, pertussis, and tetanus had come into wide use by then, and typhoid and flu vaccines for children were gaining traction, too. But because mumps was "mild" in children and none of its vaccines offered more than a year of protection, they should be used only in those for whom an attack of mumps would be "undesirable" due to other clinical conditions, they argued.[62] When the first vaccines came to market over the next few years, the American Medical Association issued a slightly less conservative recommendation, endorsing mumps vaccination to prevent widespread epidemics among children in "orphanages or boarding schools" and for adults in "closely segregated populations."[63] But at an AAP panel three years later, Werner Henle and colleagues shared the view that for children, the disease was still preferable to the vaccine.

This position was disseminated through medical texts like Saul Krugman and Robert Ward's 1958 *Infectious Diseases of Children*; because mumps was "usually benign," and because delaying infection could lead to more severe disease, no special action should be taken for the child at risk, they wrote.[64] But because of the prominence of mumps orchitis, the very question of vaccinating children raised the question of which children the disease threatened: girls or boys. Krugman and Ward described mumps as a disease that affected both sexes "equally," even as they sought to erase widespread fear of eventual sexual impotence and sterility in boys. "The extensive experience with mumps orchitis in World Wars I and II failed to demonstrate that impotence and sterility are important consequences," they wrote.[65] And yet the growing medical emphasis on mumps as a disease of boys and girls may have had unintended consequences. "By mistake, cold packs were used on the neck," the parent of a daughter with mumps wrote to physician Theodore Van Dellen. "Will this result in sterility?" Van Dellen replied simply: "No."[66]

Meanwhile, mumps received its most explicit treatment in the medical literature yet as a threat to men's procreative ability, even as new studies confirmed it posed little procreative risk to women.[67] The most comprehensive review of mumps since Comby's, published by Swedish scientist Bengt Lambert in 1951, found that men who had suffered mumps orchitis had a lower marriage rate, less sex, and fewer children; a few qualified as "eunuchoids" for their "feminine bodily habitus," including sparse body hair, small penis, and "fatty breasts."[68] As U.S. birthrates climbed and fatherhood became a widely presumed and highly valued role in the context of the Cold War, this new evidence seemed to confirm mumps as a threat to "family fever"; mumps could strip a man of procreation as an indication of his "potency and ability to provide."[69] In the meantime, familiar patterns of popular representation persisted: men's cases made the news when they struck sports teams, from the Dodgers to the Rams.[70] For women, mumps was still a means of connection to children and the home, as it was for the Culver City mayor forced to resign to take care of her mumps-stricken children, or actress Shirley Temple Black, who caught mumps from her son.[71] As vaccine research accelerated in the 1950s, gendered depictions of mumps' significance in adults persisted even as sex-based etiological differences among children were deemphasized.

In 1963, virologist Maurice Hilleman, head of Virus and Cell Biology at the burgeoning pharmaceutical company Merck, responded to his daughter's mumps infection by swabbing her throat and using the virus to develop a live-attenuated mumps vaccine. Hilleman's vaccine, dubbed Mumpsvax, was twice as protective and offered twice the duration of immunity as the war-developed vaccines. But physicians and the public greeted it with familiar ambivalence when it was licensed for use in 1967. Prominent newspapers buried the news. Medical journals questioned the need. The *New England Journal of Medicine*'s editors pointed out that mumps' complications had long been overstated.[72] Editors of the *Lancet* noted that mumps was far less urgent than other targets of vaccination, namely, smallpox and polio.[73] By this time, the baby boom had proved American men's procreative ability, and new health concerns for men, especially heart disease and hypertension, loomed much larger.[74] For American men in a time of peace, mumps was of little concern.[75]

Merck struggled, initially, to find a market for the vaccine. Early ads featured an image of a young father and his preteen son riding bicycles with the text: "To help avoid the discomfort, the inconvenience—and the possibility of complications: Mumpsvax."[76] Sales took off only after Merck introduced a combined vaccine, which protected against mumps along with measles and rubella, in 1971, and researchers began to demonstrate several years of protection, not just two.[77] Federal vaccination recommendations, which evolved in direct response to the development of the combined vaccine, played an important role. In 1967, a federal committee recommended the vaccine for boys approaching puberty, men who had not yet had the mumps, and children in institutions where mumps outbreaks could be "particularly disruptive."[78] The committee's 1972 recommendations, revised in light of the combined vaccine and reports that the mumps component offered four years of protection, stated that anyone over the age of one could be vaccinated but that mumps vaccination should not take priority over "more essential" health concerns.[79] Despite these tepid endorsements, the vaccination of children took off. By 1974, 40 percent of U.S. children had been vaccinated against mumps, and the number of annual cases had fallen to fewer than 60,000.[80] The federal committee made yet another revision in 1977, stating that "large scale production" of combined vaccines had made mumps vaccination "a practical component of routine immunization activities" and that mumps vaccination was "recommended for all children at any age after 12 months."[81] In 1981, the United States saw just under 5,000 cases of mumps, an all-time low.[82]

Mumps' inclusion in the combined measles-mumps-rubella (MMR) vaccine is one of several factors that explain how a vaccine originally pursued as a means of protecting men in war very quickly became a readily accepted vaccine for all children in a time of peace. Federal support for measles eradication spawned high-profile national measles immunization campaigns in the 1960s and a generation of laws making measles vaccination mandatory for children in the 1970s.[83] A nationwide rubella epidemic in the mid-1960s had spread panic about the infection and its ability to cause birth defects; support for its new vaccine came easily. Thanks to the combined MMR vaccine, mumps vaccination benefited from support for rubella and measles prevention, but its acceptance was not automatic or unquestioned. Shortly after Mumpsvax's approval, Centers for Disease Control and Prevention (CDC) epidemiologist Adolf Karchmer gave a talk in which he acknowledged large gaps in scientific understanding of mumps. Its seeming preference for boys, the risk of sterility, and its nervous system complications were still poorly understood, he said, and the agency was concerned about the prospect of eliminating the disease in children only to leave a population of adults, namely men, at risk down the line.[84] The CDC subsequently placed mumps on the list of nationally notifiable diseases and asked state health departments to inform the agency of outbreaks its epidemiologists could use to study the disease. The studies focused exclusively on children, thanks to epidemics in homes for orphans, the deaf, and the "mentally retarded," and a detailed picture of mumps in children soon emerged. It threatened both sexes. It required "intimate" contact to spread, took more than two weeks to incubate, and caused few complications, although orchitis did occur among older boys. Infected children also carried the disease from institutions into communities.[85]

In the meantime, published reports on the mumps vaccine by Hilleman and others had begun to emphasize the nervous system complications first suggested in nineteenth-century reports. "Mumps is a common childhood disease that may be severely and even permanently crippling when it involves the brain . . ." began a series of articles that Hilleman and colleagues published in prominent journals.[86] The articles tied a non-sex-specific, severe complication of mumps to all children, downplaying the disease's severe consequences in adults. This framing linked mumps to the tragic specter of the recent rubella epidemic, which had led to children with birth defects including deafness and "mental retardation"—complications that increasingly became cited in connection with mumps. Mumps' framing as a cause of deafness or brain damage was particularly resonant at a time when, as Leslie Reagan has shown, a child's impairment had physical, social, and financial consequences for the entire family.[87] Polio, measles, and rubella all threatened children and their families, with the specter of costly, isolating, and stigmatizing disability. Their vaccines, all developed and recommended (or required) for children in the 1950s and 1960s, promised protection from this threat and forged a narrative about the modern vaccine's role in safeguarding a healthy, productive, and "normal" middle-class existence. The emphasis on mumps' nervous system complications—the only complications made reportable when the CDC made mumps notifiable—helped weave mumps into this narrative, too.

As these risks came to be cited in the scientific literature, mumps' threat to adults, namely men, began to fade in professional and popular discourse. Mumps' orchitis risk, meanwhile, wove the disease into a separate narrative. As a vaccine administered to all children in order to protect expecting mothers and their babies, the rubella vaccine, according to Reagan, "represented a historic transformation in the expectations surrounding a vaccine."[88] It was used not to give direct benefit to the recipient but to protect "the nation's future citizens."[89] The childhood mumps vaccine belongs in this category as well. It was the opposite-sex corollary to the rubella vaccine, given to all children to ensure boys' gendered role in producing future citizens and in serving, more specifically, as the nation's future men, soldiers, laborers, and fathers. In this sense, the promotion of mumps vaccination in all children anticipated the much later use of HPV vaccination to prepare children for a presumed future as heterosexual adults, as Laura Mamo has shown elsewhere.[90]

Mumps' transformation from a severe disease of men to a severe disease of children was swift after the vaccine's approval. When Mumpsvax was licensed in 1967, newspapers described it as a "mild" disease that was "relatively harmless" and for which "serious complications" were "unusual."[91] By the end of the 1970s, newspapers were describing mumps as a "scary" disease that could cause deafness and "take the edge off a child's intelligence."[92] The reporting mirrored a shift in government and medical sources. A CDC immunization recommendation from Mumpsvax's early days described meningeal swelling and deafness as "rare" and sterility as "very rare." A late-seventies brochure published by the Department of Health, Education, and Welfare, however, said simply, "Mumps can cause deafness, diabetes, and brain damage. It can make boys sterile."[93] By the late 1970s, mumps' transformation to a severe threat to all children, if still a unique threat to boys, was complete.

Two hundred years of mumps' historical epidemiology reflects gendered patterns of social organization. Urbanization, compulsory schooling, workforce patterns, military activity, women's employment outside the home, the institutionalization of children from orphans to the intellectually impaired—all gave shape to the patterns of who contracted mumps and when in the prevaccine era. Mumps had two competing identities in this era, as both a mild disease of children, especially boys, and as a severe disease of men. These identities persisted until the development of a vaccine that offered lasting protection, licensed in a team of peace and prosperity in the United States. The timing of the mumps vaccine and the combined MMR vaccine's approval made mumps a severe disease of children, transferring its long-known risks to adolescent and adult men onto children and presenting them as equivalent to a long list of additional risks not nearly as well understood or quantified. The deployment of the vaccine, still in use today, thus erased questions of gender and sex, even as these were deeply embedded in the vaccine's long development and perceptions of the disease's severity for the preceding two hundred years.

Notes

1. Robert Hamilton, "An Account of a Distemper, by the Common People in England Vulgarly Called the Mumps," *Transactions of the Royal Society of Edinburgh* 2, no. 2 (1790): 59–72.
2. Elena Conis, "'Do We Really Need Hepatitis B on the Second Day of Life?' Vaccination Mandates and Shifting Representations of Hepatitis B," *Journal of Medical Humanities* 32, no. 2 (2011): 155–66; Keith Wailoo et al., eds, *Three Shots at Prevention: The HPV Vaccine and the Politics of Medicine's Simple Solutions* (Baltimore: Johns Hopkins University Press, 2012).
3. Hamilton, "An Account."
4. Hamilton, "An Account."
5. A. L. Peirson, "Observations upon Parotitis, or Mumps," *New England Journal of Medicine and Surgery* 13, no. 2 (1824): 116.
6. "Children's Diseases—A Suggestion," *Chicago Tribune*, July 30, 1861, 4.
7. "Coast Notes," *San Francisco Chronicle*, February 27, 1884, 4; "A Cat Has the Mumps," *Chicago Daily Tribune*, March 15, 1879, 13; "For the Ladies," *San Francisco Chronicle*, May 9, 1880, 6.
8. A. B. Isham, "Article V: Parotiditis, or Mumps," *American Journal of the Medical Sciences* 9, no. 1 (1878): 532.
9. Isham, "Article V."
10. Constance Beerbohm, "England's Queen," *San Francisco Chronicle*, November 10, 1889, 1.

11. See, for example, "Movements and Doings at Camp Douglas," *Chicago Tribune*, February 26, 1862, 4.

12. Drew Gilpin Faust, *This Republic of Suffering: Death and the American Civil War* (New York: Vintage Books, 2009).

13. Isham, "Article V."

14. "General Notes," *New York Times*, March 11, 1881, 4; "Star Chamber Findings," *Washington Post*, November 25, 1879, 1; "The School Ship St. Mary's," *New York Times*, December 3, 1880, 8; "Indiana: Mumps in an Orphan Asylum," *Chicago Daily Tribune*, March 11, 1884, 11. On gendered expectations of men in this period, see Robert Griswold, *Fatherhood in America: A History* (New York: Basic Books, 1993); E. Anthony Rotundo, *American Manhood: Transformations in American Masculinity from the Revolution to the Modern Era* (New York: Basic Books, 1994).

15. P. M. Walsh Mecray, "Some Notes on the Bacteriology of Mumps," *Medical Record* 50, no. 13 (1896): 440–42.

16. "Students Down with the Mumps," *Chicago Daily Tribune*, March 6, 1986, 3.

17. For a summary, see Comby, "Mumps," in Thomas L. Stedman, ed., *Twentieth Century Practice: An International Encyclopedia of Modern Medical Science* (New York: William Wood, 1898), 555–603.

18. R. Percy Smith, "Insanity Following Mumps," *Lancet* 134, no. 3441 (1889): 265.

19. Mark S. Micale, *Hysterical Men: The Hidden History of Male Nervous Illness* (Cambridge, MA: Harvard University Press, 2009), 57; Rotundo, *American Manhood*, 6.

20. "Because He Had the Mumps," *Washington Post*, June 25, 1881, 1.

21. "Affected by Mumps," *New York Times*, April 1, 1884, 2; "Undertones," *San Francisco Chronicle*, April 13, 1884, 7.

22. F. D. Haldeman, "Unusual Metastasis in Mumps," *Journal of the American Medical Association* 8, no. 20 (1887): 543–45.

23. Mecray, "Some Notes."

24. Comby, "Mumps."

25. Micale, *Hysterical Men*, 49.

26. Rotundo, *American Manhood*, 222.

27. Comby, "Mumps," 578.

28. "American Soldiers Are Captured by Germans," *San Francisco Chronicle*, February 10, 1918, 1.

29. "Americans Shifted in Trenches Again," *New York Times*, November 14, 1917, 3.

30. "How to Keep Well," *Chicago Daily Tribune*, October 13, 1920, 8.

31. Russell L. Haden, "The Bacteriology of Mumps: Report of Findings at Camp Lee," *American Journal of the Medical Sciences* 158, no. 5 (1919): 698–702.

32. C. G. Sinclair, "Mumps: Epidemiology and Influence of the Disease on the Non-Effective Rate in the Army," *Military Surgeon* 50 (June 1922): 626.

33. Sinclair, "Mumps"; Bengt Lambert, *The Frequency of Mumps and of Mumps Orchitis and the Consequences for Sexuality and Fertility* (Uppsala, Sweden: State Institute of Human Genetics and Race Biology, 1951).

34. Sinclair, "Mumps."

35. Beth Linker, *War's Waste: Rehabilitation in World War I America* (Chicago: University of Chicago Press, 2011), 28.

36. Ralph LaRossa, *The Modernization of Fatherhood: A Social and Political History* (Chicago: University of Chicago Press, 1997).

37. Robert Griswold, *Fatherhood in America: A History* (New York: Basic Books, 1993); "Dr. A Wilberforce Williams," *Chicago Defender*, March 28, 1925, A8.

38. Philip Lovell, "Care of the Body: The Coefficient of Bug Killing," *Los Angeles Times*, October 6, 1940, I17.
39. Philip Lovell, "Care of the Body: Mumps," *Los Angeles Times*, March 11, 1928, K26.
40. Irving Cutter, "How to Keep Well: Mumps or Parotitis," *Washington Post*, December 23, 1934, R7; Irving Cutter, "Today's Health Talk," *Washington Post*, January 9, 1937, 12.
41. Logan Clendening, "Today's Health Talk," *Washington Post*, February 22, 1937, 13.
42. Irving Cutter, "How to Keep Well," *Chicago Daily Tribune*, January 15, 1938, 12.
43. Logan Clendening, "Today's Health Talk," *Washington Post*, January 17, 1938, 11.
44. Ernest Goodpasture and Claud D. Johnson, "An Investigation of the Etiology of Mumps," *Journal of Experimental Medicine* 59 (1934): 1–19.
45. Ernest Goodpasture and Claud D. Johnson, "The Etiology of Mumps," *American Journal of Epidemiology* 21, no. 1 (1935): 46–57.
46. "How to Keep Well," *Washington Post*, March 2, 1925, 12.
47. Aims C. McGuiness and Edward A. Gall, "Mumps at Army Camps in 1943," *War Medicine* 5, no. 2 (1944): 95–104.
48. "Disease Rate of U.S. Troops at Record Low," *Chicago Daily Tribune*, October 17, 1943, 25.
49. Marshall Andrews, "331 Officers Recommended for Promotion," *Washington Post*, March 19, 1941, 30.
50. McGuiness and Gall, "Mumps at Army Camps."
51. Joseph Stokes Jr., "History of the Commission on Measles and Mumps," 1946, Stanhope Bayne-Jones Papers, National Library of Medicine.
52. McGuiness and Gall, "Mumps at Army Camps."
53. A. W. Frankland, "Mumps Meningo-Encephalitis," *British Medical Journal* 2, no. 4201 (1941): 48–49.
54. James P. Halcrow and Ian Wang, "Mumps Meningo-Encephalitis and Orchitis," *British Medical Journal* 1, no. 4404 (1945): 770–71.
55. "Mumps Serum Aids Monkeys, Tested on Man," *Washington Post*, November 27, 1946, 4.
56. "Communicable Disease Toll Nearly Doubled for State," *Los Angeles Times*, May 21, 1942, 26.
57. "Government Move Demanded to Save BWI Workers Lives," *New York Amsterdam News*, March 10, 1945, 2A.
58. Karl Habel, "Vaccination of Human Beings against Mumps: Vaccine Administered at the Start of an Epidemic," *American Journal of Hygiene* 54, no. 3 (1951): 295–311.
59. "Vaccine May Yield Preventive for Mumps," *New York Times*, April 3, 1946, 26.
60. "Vaccine May Yield Preventive for Mumps."
61. Gertrude Henle and Werner Henle, "Studies on the Prevention of Mumps," *Pediatrics* 8, no. 1 (1951): 1–4.
62. Henle and Henle, "Studies."
63. "Council on Drugs," *Journal of the American Medical Association* 164, no. 8 (1957): 874–75.
64. Saul Krugman and Robert Ward, *Infectious Diseases of Children* (St. Louis, MO: C. V. Mosby Company, 1958), 152–64.
65. Krugman and Ward, *Infectious Diseases.*
66. Theodore Van Dellen, "How to Keep Well: Dog Bites and Rabies," *Chicago Daily Tribune*, April 16, 1948, 16.
67. Harold A. Schwartz, "Mumps in Pregnancy," *American Journal of Obstetrics and Gynecology* 60 (1950): 875–76.

68. Lambert, "The Frequency of Mumps."

69. Elaine Tyler May, *Homeward Bound: American Families in the Cold War Era* (New York: Basic Books, 2008), 151.

70. Roscoe McGowen, "Mumps Increase Woes of Dodgers," *New York Times*, March 16, 1957, 16; Frank Finch, "Ram Center Laid Low with Mumps," *Los Angeles Times*, December 21, 1955, C1.

71. Cordell Hicks, "Mumps, Mumps, Mumps Replace Mayor Duty," *Los Angeles Times*, May 27, 1959, B1; Associated Press, "Has the Mumps," *Chicago Daily Tribune*, September 22, 1955, 5.

72. "Mumps Vaccine: More Information Needed," *New England Journal of Medicine* 278, no. 5 (1968): 275–76.

73. "Vaccination against Mumps," *Lancet* 292, no. 7576 (1968): 1022–23.

74. Elianne Riska, "From Type A Man to the Hardy Man: Masculinity and Health," *Sociology of Health & Illness* 24, no. 3 (2002): 347–58; Tracy Penny Light, "'Healthy' Men Make Good Fathers: Masculine Health and the Family in 1950s America," in *Inventing the Modern American Family*, edited by Isabel Heinemann (New York: Campus Verlag, 2012), 105–23.

75. Elena Conis, *Vaccine Nation* (Chicago: University of Chicago Press, 2015), 66.

76. Merck, "The First Live Mumps Vaccine," *British Medical Journal* 2, no. 5910 (April 13, 1971), front matter.

77. Robert E. Weibel, Eugene B. Buynak, Joseph Stokes, and Maurice Hilleman, "Persistence of Immunity Four Years following Jeryl Lynn Strain Live Mumps Virus Vaccine," *Pediatrics* 45, no. 5 (1970): 821–26.

78. Advisory Committee on Immunization Practices, "Recommendation of the Public Health Service Advisory Committee on Immunization Practices," *Morbidity and Mortality Weekly Report* 16, no. 51 (1967): 430–31.

79. "Mumps Vaccine," *Morbidity and Mortality Weekly Report* 21, suppl. (1972): 13–14.

80. Jennifer Hamborsky, Andrew Kroger, and Charles Wolfe, *Epidemiology and Prevention of Vaccine-Preventable Diseases*, 13th ed. (Washington, D.C.: Public Health Foundation, 2015).

81. "Mumps Vaccine," *Morbidity and Mortality Weekly Report* 26, no. 48 (1977): 393–94.

82. Hamborsky et al., *Epidemiology and Prevention*.

83. Conis, *Vaccine Nation*, 50–61.

84. Adolf Karchmer, "Mumps: A Review of Surveillance, Vaccine Development, and Recommendations for Use," Folder: Paper for Immunization Conference, Box 343357, National Archives at Atlanta, Record Group 442.

85. Conis, *Vaccine Nation*, 73–74.

86. Robert E. Weibel, Joseph Stokes, Eugene Buynak, James E. Whitman, and Maurice Hilleman, "Live, Attenuated Mumps-Virus Vaccine," *New England Journal of Medicine* 276, no. 5 (1967): 245–51; Joseph Stokes, Robert Weibel, Eugene Buynak, and Maurice Hilleman, "Live Attenuated Mumps Virus Vaccine: II. Early Clinical Studies," *Pediatrics* 39, no. 3 (1967): 363–71.

87. Leslie Reagan, *Dangerous Pregnancies: Mothers, Disabilities, and Abortion in Modern America* (Berkeley: University of California Press, 2010), 68.

88. Reagan, *Dangerous Pregnancies*, 181.

89. Reagan, *Dangerous Pregnancies*, 181.

90. Laura Mamo, Amber Nelson, and Aleia Clark, "Producing and Protecting Risky Girlhoods," in *Three Shots*, edited by Wailoo et al., 123.

Chapter 8

Weight, Height, and the Gendering of Nutritional Assessment

A. R. Ruis

"My daughter's school weighed the entire class yesterday," tweeted the American pediatrician Clay Jones on January 9, 2019. "She comes home asking if she weighs too much because other girls who weigh 100 pounds were complaining about being fat. They all compared weights. I am furious. What the hell were they thinking?"[1] Jones's concern was not only that of a parent but also of a health care professional. "I take care of patients with eating disorders. They can often tell you when they developed concerns about their weight. They can tell you the day," he continued in a subsequent tweet. "It's incredibly irresponsible for a school to focus on weight at all, and so much worse to do it in a group setting."[2]

While group weighing of children is not a common practice in American schools today, it was nearly ubiquitous a century ago. "Group competition based upon the record of height and weight," wrote the pediatrician and nutrition specialist L. Emmett Holt in 1922, was one of the simplest and "most potent" ways to interest children in their nutritional health, and he argued that children's weights should be regularly recorded and hung on the classroom wall for all to see.[3] By 1920, the Wisconsin State Board of Health had begun to include instructions for the regular weighing and measuring of children under "Suggestions for School Boards," confident that "the day is not far distant when scales will come to be considered as essential a part of schoolroom equipment as the blackboard, map, and globe have been."[4] Schools typically weighed and measured children on a monthly basis, and children who consistently failed to gain weight or who fell significantly below some standard for "normal" weight were considered malnourished (see figure 8.1).

91. "Mumps Vaccine Now Ready for Public," *Los Angeles Sentinel*, March 28, 1968, Associated Press, "Vaccine for Mumps Licensed," *Washington Post*, January 5, 196 A1; Harold Schmeck, "A Mumps Vaccine Is Licensed by the US," *New York Time* January 5, 1968, 72.

92. See, for example, Midge L. Schildkraut, "The New Threat to Your Children's Health *Good Housekeeping*, August 1978, 219–20.

93. U.S. Department of Health, Education, and Welfare, *Protect Your Child* (Washington D.C.: Office of Human Development Services, 1978).

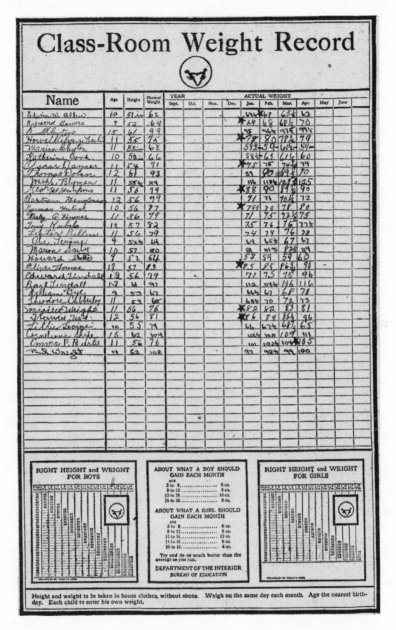

Figure 8.1. "One of these records should hang on every schoolroom wall." Sample record of schoolchildren's age, height, and monthly weights, issued by the U.S. Bureau of Education in partnership with the Child Health Organization. The starred entries identify students whose weight measurements exceeded the "normal weight" for their age and height. The tables in the lower left and lower right give the normal weights by height and age for boys and girls, respectively, while the table in the lower center indicates how much weight boys and girls of different ages should gain each month. Source: L. Emmett Holt, *Your Opportunity in the Schools* (U.S. Bureau of Education, Health Education No. 9, 1922), 12.

While the scale did not ultimately become an "essential" feature of U.S. classrooms, it has long been a central tool of diagnostic medicine and public health surveillance alike.[5] Weight is perhaps chief among the basic indicators of health, but it promotes a discourse of self-knowledge and self-management as the mechanism through which a disciplined body becomes (or remains) a healthy body.[6] The idea that simple anthropometric measurements such as weight can be used for early detection and ongoing prevention of potential nutritional issues, which are characterized by complex causal frameworks and numerous interaction effects, remains an alluring one.

Yet Jones's tweets also reflect the historical processes through which measuring and interpreting children's weights to assess their nutritional status were explicitly and implicitly gendered. On one hand, it is perhaps not surprising that it is the girls who "were complaining about being fat" and who "compared weights." Although weight was constructed as an objective metric of nutritional status during the early twentieth century, the uses to which scales and their readings were put reflected deeply ingrained beliefs about biological and social differences between boys and girls (and also among different racial and ethnic groups). Health programs designed to help undernourished children often disseminated different strategies for boys and girls. Moreover, even as skepticism of weight as a valid measure of nutrition mounted during the 1930s and 1940s, those critiques did not seriously interrogate whether separate standards for boys and girls were even appropriate.

On the other hand, weighing and measuring children in schools and other public health contexts was increasingly criticized by physicians on the grounds that such measurements, divorced from physical examination and longitudinal observation, were of limited diagnostic value. Yet this pitted predominantly male pediatricians against the mostly female school teachers, nurses, and dietitians who implemented such programs. While this conflict emerged in part from the efforts of pediatricians to assume well-child care as part of their professional purview,[7] it also reflected concern that too much diagnostic authority was being ceded to those who were not "trained medical men."[8]

This chapter briefly explores several dimensions along which gender was operant in the emergence of public health nutrition in the early twentieth century, a formative period in the development of nutrition science, pediatrics, and school-based health services more generally in the United States.[9] The nutrition class—a comprehensive program for undernourished children offered in dispensaries, schools, and other contexts during the 1910s and 1920s—forms a focal case study for exploring how public health nutrition initiatives engendered conceptions of nutrition differently for boys and girls and how such programs revealed gender-based fault lines in the professionalization of public health nutrition.

The nutrition class, sometimes called the nutrition clinic, was designed to help undernourished children achieve and maintain good health through a combination of routine medical examination and care, supplemental feeding, instruction in foods and nutrition, and social work. The first nutrition class was conducted in 1908 by William R. P. Emerson, professor of pediatrics at Tufts Medical School, who selected fifteen "of the weakest and most poorly nourished children out of the four or five thousand patients" who visited the Children's Department of the Boston Dispensary to test the theory that "directions of hygiene and diet could be given to the group in much less time and much more effectively than to each one individually."[10] After a complete physical examination, each child received a notebook to record the details of his or her diet, exercise, personal hygiene, and sleep, and a social worker visited their homes and reported on the quality of the living conditions. Emerson then spoke with the children and their parents as a group, giving lectures on general hygiene, diet, care of the teeth, physical activity, and rest.

Over the following year, the children and their parents attended the nutrition class every Saturday morning for one hour. Emerson and his assistants weighed the children as they arrived and seated them according to how much weight they had gained. The primary method of instruction involved the public examination of each child's notebook and weight record and subsequent discussion of the causes of weight loss or gain in each case. This competitive model was intended to motivate children to gain weight. Presenting health as a game to be won was a common tactic in the "new" health education paradigm that emerged during the Progressive era. Rather than the simple, didactic methods of the nineteenth-century monitorial system—consisting of lessons in basic anatomy and physiology and personal care—the new health education utilized child-designed materials, games, stories, songs, pageants, and other mechanisms to entice children to see their health as the outcome of vigilant efforts to monitor and improve oneself.[11] The nutrition class focused on weight, as weight (and its rate of change) was widely considered one of the best metrics of nutritional status and thus of overall health, but children also received instruction in exercise, rest, personal hygiene, and other aspects of self-care.

After the first year of Emerson's pilot nutrition class, eight children "graduated" by coming up to normal weight for their age and height and by improving in overall health; all of the remaining seven children had improved, but they were still below normal weight. Emerson's initial study provided the model for conducting nutrition classes, and over the next two decades, the class method gained popularity with school and public health authorities.

The nutrition class model was adopted widely. For example, the Elizabeth McCormick Memorial Fund, which was established "to promote the health, happiness and general welfare of children," secured the approval of the Chicago Board of Education to set up nutrition classes based on Emerson's model in eight public elementary schools and three high schools in the city, as well as at two private schools in the suburbs. The Fund employed a physician and eight nutrition workers, most of whom were dietitians with social work training and all of whom were women, and the Board of Education supplied a physician and three visiting teachers. The physicians performed the initial physical examinations (and any follow-up exams deemed necessary), while the nutrition workers conducted the classes and made home visits. The classes were run exactly as laid out by Emerson and with comparable results. Many of the children gained 1 to 1.5 pounds per week after beginning the class.[12]

Emerson's method became popular in part because it emphasized individual self-care and promoted a pedagogical solution to structural health problems—ignorance, not poverty, was widely regarded as the most important root cause of endemic malnourishment—and in part because it promised to address the shockingly high rates of preventable morbidity revealed by regular school medical inspection and the military medical exams conducted during World War I. But Emerson also made health a competitive activity by assigning to weight not only the measurement of nutritional status but also adherence to lessons on diet and personal care. Those lessons were based not only on knowledge of nutrition science and his experience as a pediatrician but also on gender-based assumptions about how to motivate children. "All girls want to be attractive and beautiful. They also want to do as other girls do, dance, swim and play tennis," Emerson wrote in 1914 of his approach to encouraging children to change their diets. "Every boy wants to be athletic. The desire to play baseball and football can always be aroused in him sufficiently to cause him to do almost anything to gain a good physical condition for that purpose."[13] Lucy Oppen gave similar advice to classroom teachers. "Every girl desires to be beautiful, and every boy desires to be strong and athletic," she wrote in a widely circulated pamphlet published by the U.S. Bureau of Education in 1919, "and the wise teacher will build on these natural interests of the children, and inspire them to do the things which will result in physical beauty and strength."[14]

This framing was even more pronounced in food advertisements, and the new health education borrowed liberally from the toolkit of product marketing.

For example, breakfast cereals such as those produced by National Oats and Quaker Oats sold mothers on the idea of robust, active (white) boys and rosy-cheeked, bright-eyed (white) girls. In the early twentieth century, when an advertisement emphasized the benefits of cereal consumption for physical development or performance, the imagery typically depicted a boy playing sports or engaging in other athletic endeavors. Similarly, when the advertisement emphasized the benefits of cereal consumption for appearance—especially "rosy cheeks"—the imagery typically depicted a girl, still and often framed as if she were a cameo. National Oats, for example, presented contrasting images of boys and girls under the slogan "makes kids husky." A National Oats advertisement that appeared in a 1919 issue of *The Designer* (figure 8.2) shows a grinning boy kicking a football while his companions struggle to keep up with him. (They, presumably, did not have National Oats cereal for breakfast.) When National Oats ads depicted girls (see figure 8.3), their "huskiness" was communicated not as an athletic capacity but as a trait of beauty or comportment. The girl sits, like a porcelain doll, merely watching as her brother(?) performs a

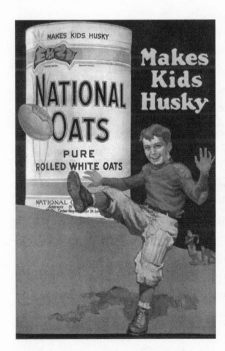
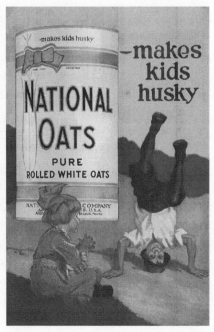

Figure 8.2. National Oats advertisement. Source: *The Designer* (November 1919), 60.

Figure 8.3. National Oats advertisement. Source: *Ladies' Home Journal* (September 1920), 162.

gymnastic feat. In another advertisement (not pictured), a boy flexes his arm as a girl squeezes and admires his bicep.[15] With his other thumb, he points back to the can of National Oats.

Advertisements for food products that were intended for children routinely constructed boys as active and athletic and girls as passive and demure. Although accompanying text (when included) typically referenced "children" and a wider spectrum of advantages to consuming the advertised product, the imagery clearly delineated those advantages along gendered lines, similar to those of nutrition classes.

While the nutrition class and other nutrition improvement initiatives— including extension work, little mothers' clubs, well-baby clinics, better baby contests, school meals, and other hallmarks of Progressive-era children's health work—were clearly steeped in the eugenic language of bodily improvement and racial purity, they did not typically advance an explicitly eugenic, racialized, or nationalist agenda.[16] Indeed, nutritionists often pushed back against eugenic frameworks even as they reified many core eugenic tenets. For example, Ellen Richards's 1910 book, *Euthenics, the Science of Controllable Environment*, urged a shift in focus from hereditary to environmental factors to address nutrition health problems, and nutritionists embraced the idea that poverty and ignorance were the most significant root causes of malnourishment.[17] Although some acknowledged that ignorance was a problem irrespective of class or race, immigrants, "Negroes," "Mexicans," and others were often singled out for the purported depths of their ignorance. "There is great difficulty [doing nutrition work in Negro schools]," wrote two home economists from Missouri, "because many of the parents are careless, unreliable, indifferent and ignorant. Workers with these people must be patient, tireless and must expect slow results."[18] Euthenics did not reduce racism and placed perhaps more emphasis on individual responsibility, which easily accommodated racist beliefs. Noting that communicable diseases were declining while "troubles under personal control," such as heart disease, were increasingly prevalent, Richards argued that "such results of improper personal living . . . show the attitude of mind of the great mass of the people, 'Let us eat and drink and be merry, what if we do die tomorrow!'"[19] And the burden of responsibility for poor personal choices, especially the poor choices of children, fell largely on mothers.

As Rachel Moran has shown in her work on the rise of the "advisory state," public health nutrition programs were emblematic of a shift in health policy that leveraged advertising, quantification, volunteerism, and spectacle to entice individuals to self-monitor and self-improve.[20] In addition to poverty and ignorance, nutritionists often focused on a "lack of home control" as a key cause of children's malnourishment, and the advisory state focused considerable effort on mothers to exert this control over their children.[21] Yet this application of soft power also necessitated a certain ecumenical approach to public health nutrition. It was much easier and more effective, for example, to convince children and their families to modify elements of their diet and regimen than to replace them wholesale, and it was important that everyone learn how to eat for health, not merely satiety or pleasure. This led to broad acceptance of dietary heterogeneity based on race, ethnicity, and religion—as long as those diets could be made to meet scientific standards for nutritional content—and to recommendations that boys as well as girls be educated in foods and nutrition.

Yet underlying this approach to nutrition improvement was the idea that boys needed to grow into strong, healthy workers, and girls needed to grow into competent, healthy mothers and caregivers, regardless of race or ethnicity. For example, the story of Theodore Roosevelt's bodily transformation from an effeminate New York state assemblyman to the Cowboy of the Dakotas was included in nutrition health lessons in order to motivate boys to pursue strength through proper diet, vigorous exercise, and adequate rest. In one nutrition class, "interest in Roosevelt and his determination to overcome his weakness of body was keen."[22] It is not clear from extant sources whether similarly famous figures were used to motivate girls, but the implicit messaging was clear: building the nation meant building the body, and the future strength of the nation was predicated on the robustness of its children.

This tension between treating boys and girls as having the same basic need—to consume a diet that would support optimal growth and health—but fundamentally different social roles was often resolved as children aged. "It is well to enlist the help of every boy and girl in the grammar grades of the school" in meal service, argued the author of a 1920 pamphlet on school nutrition distributed by the U.S. Bureau of Education. "Both boys and girls delight" in this work, but "an upper grade pupil, *preferably a girl*, may for a week at a time act as manager of the volunteer helpers" (emphasis added).[23] Similarly, nutrition work begun in 1917 by the Association for Improving the Conditions of the Poor in the schools and clinics of New York City's Columbus Hill district, which was "peopled largely by Negroes," enlisted older girls to assist young children in the nutrition classes. Girls who showed "improvement in nutrition and general health while members of the nutrition class" were enrolled in the Little Mothers Club. "Each girl has chosen a malnourished child about six years of age and is learning how to weigh the child and to teach him how to form good health habits."[24]

While nutritionists and educators were advocating for boys to take domestic science classes, formerly offered only to girls, older girls were nonetheless socialized into the role of household manager and caregiver. That is, as children aged, they were increasingly guided into gendered understandings of their roles in maintaining good nutrition: boys needed strong muscles to meet the needs of a growing industrial economy, and girls needed to learn how to properly feed and care for their future families.

With its combination of supplemental feeding, education, social work, and competition, the nutrition class method typically led to gains in weight and improvements in children's health.[25] Follow-up studies indicated that while children did not retain all the benefits of the class once they left, they maintained better nutritional health than children who had never been enrolled in nutrition classes. Furthermore, evidence suggested that the lessons learned in nutrition classes were passed informally to friends and family.

Yet despite its successes, the nutrition class model was largely abandoned by the early 1930s. While the onset of the Great Depression was perhaps the most acute challenge to the nutrition class model—nutrition education was at best an anemic antidote to abject hunger and collapsing agricultural markets—that model was already declining in the late 1920s. This decline stemmed in part from criticism about the utility of anthropometry to assess nutrition status and in part from increasing opposition to individualized public health nutrition programs from physicians and the American Medical Association.

Although standard weight tables of varying quality were available beginning in the late nineteenth century, physicians had used them primarily to chart the growth, development, and overall health of children whom they examined on a regular basis. After World War I, with the rapid expansion of public health nutrition efforts, such tables were increasingly used to determine, at any given time, the deviation from "normal" weight. Health workers generally used either 7 percent or 10 percent of normal weight for height (or height and age) to mark the boundary between malnourishment and relative health. Use of weight tables in this way was so simple as to require "no expert medical knowledge," according to the U.S. Bureau of Education. "The weight of the child and his rate of gain usually tell the story."[26] This made it possible for nearly anyone to weigh and measure children in a range of public health contexts.

Physicians, however, came to regard such efforts as infringing on their professional prerogatives. Assistant Surgeon General Taliaferro Clark criticized weighing and measuring as conducted by people with "limited training and experience in health matters." He lamented that "the veriest tyro in public health work, after placing a child on a scale and noting comparative results, gravely announces the percentage of malnutrition in a given population group."[27] A physician from Chicago argued that a diagnosis of malnutrition "can be determined only by careful physical examination by an expert physician. . . . The grocery clerk system of weighing, aging and measuring must be abandoned for one conducted by trained medical men."[28] The use of standard weight charts in public health nutrition programs pitted predominantly male physicians against the mostly female nurses, teachers, and dietitians who comprised the majority of the labor force in weighing and measuring programs. The historian Jeffrey Brosco has argued that physicians, despite their initial support of anthropometric methods, ultimately rejected the use of weight charts in public health programs in order to consolidate their own authority over children's health and become the sole providers of well-child care. "The irony of promoting a simple measure of nutrition . . . was that physicians placed the diagnosis of malnutrition within the competence of non-medical personnel. Arguments by physicians that the diagnosis required an expert clinical decision," a decision only they themselves could provide, were "an important component in the emergence of pediatrics as a primary care specialty."[29]

This opposition to women-led nutrition work by male physicians emerged in part from a desire to reclaim professional ownership of nutrition and dietetics, which, over the course of the nineteenth century, had largely been ceded to folk medicine and heterodox practice. "Dietetic vocabulary and sensibilities," the historian Steven Shapin has argued, "were rapidly disappearing in official academic medicine." Although they were ultimately "replaced with the notion of chemically defined constituents and, in the case of the calorie, of the powers of those constituents," physicians had begun to focus far more attention on bacteriology and other externalized ontologies of health and illness.[30] Other professionals, however, increasingly embraced nutrition and dietetics in their public health work. Social reformers and settlement house workers employed concern about malnutrition to promote nutrition education and food relief programs for the poor, and dietitians (including many home economists) responded similarly by developing their professional identity as nutrition experts able to translate scientific research into practical diets and public education campaigns.[31] Standard weight charts became an important tool in the diagnostic and educational efforts of health professions practiced largely by women.

But many experts began to challenge not only the use of the charts to assess nutritional status but also the validity of the charts themselves. Of the thirty-six standard tables surveyed by one professor of public health in 1929, thirty-three gave different average weights for an eleven-year-old boy, with a range of 29.0 to 34.4 kg (63.8 to 75.7 lbs.); the variation in averages was even greater for girls.[32] This issue was complicated by racial disparities in height. The physiologist Henry Bowditch had noted in the 1870s that children of different races had different average heights, and both Franz Boas and Charles Davenport had published numerous studies on the effects of heredity and environment on physical and physiological attributes. By the 1920s, however, there was no consensus among anthropologists and physiologists as to the relationship of race, environment, and stature.[33] As physiologists learned more about the growth process, they came to understand that the extent and pace of growth were determined by copious factors, including heredity, geography, climate, general health, amount of exercise, diet, and even the time of the year.[34] Furthermore, aggregate data could only be reliably extended to individual cases in certain circumstances. The New York Nutrition Council's Committee on Statistics argued in 1922 that "there is no warrant for assuming that the average height and weight of a large number of children is the 'normal' weight for any particular child under consideration," which undercut the primary affordance of standard weight charts for public health nutrition work.[35]

Yet while researchers called into question nearly every aspect of the standard weight charts used to assess nutritional status in schools and other public health contexts, from how they were computed to how they were applied, one assumption went notably unchallenged: the use of separate charts for boys and girls. This is not to suggest that there were no differences in development between the sexes. For example, the variance in weight for height and age among girls was greater than among boys,[36] and it was widely understood that while prepubescent boys and girls develop at about the same rate, the same could not be said for older children.[37] Yet these differences were not particularly meaningful at the coarse scale of the standard weight charts. "We have seen that there are age and sex differences," argued the statistician Raymond Franzen in 1929, based on extensive anthropometric measurements of children. "These age and sex differences tend however to occur in such a manner as to suggest that one regression equation may fit all three ages [ten, eleven, and twelve] of a sex or both sexes of an age or possibly all six age-sex groups."[38] In other words, there was no reason to believe that different weight standards were necessary for prepubescent boys and girls.

Even the most widely used standard weight chart for schoolchildren, which was produced by Columbia University professor Thomas D. Wood in 1918, gave standard weights for boys and girls that were highly similar. The relationship between height and weight was nearly identical for girls and boys (see figure 8.4), and while the rate of change in the relationship between height and weight by age was slightly different (see figure 8.5)—prepubescent girls developed at a

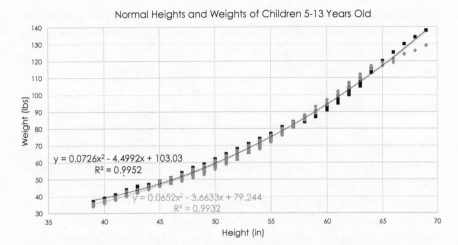

Figure 8.4. Normal heights and weights of boys (black squares) and girls (gray circles) five to thirteen years old from the most widely used table of standard weights for school-aged children. The trend lines are nearly identical for the two populations. Data source: Thomas D. Wood, *Height and Weight Table for Boys and Height and Weight Table for Girls* (Child Health Organization, 1918).

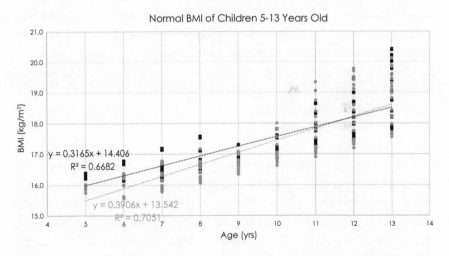

Figure 8.5. Normal body mass index (BMI) of boys (black squares) and girls (gray circles) five to thirteen years old based on the most widely used table of standard weights for school-aged children. The rate of change in BMI with age is faster for girls, but the difference is slight. Data source: *Thomas D. Wood, Height and Weight Table for Boys and Height and Weight Table for Girls* (Child Health Organization, 1918).

faster rate than prepubescent boys—the difference was not big enough to have required separate tables for classroom screening purposes. When the recommended daily allowances were first released in 1941, the recommendations for boys and girls under age thirteen were identical, providing further evidence that separate charts were likely unnecessary.[39] (For a more in-depth discussion of these issues, see the chapter by Medeiros in this volume.)

In some respects, the early twentieth-century debates over standard weight charts and who had the authority to use them were debates over the power to quantify, and yet while the allure of quantification in medicine has only grown, anthropometric measurement has generated more problems than solutions. Body mass index (BMI), for example, has all the same issues as standard weight tables, but other biometric meaures are not much better. "The numbers used to assess health," wrote the physician James Hamblin in a recent piece for *The Atlantic*, "are, for the most part, not helpful." Sure, he conceded, metrics like respiration and heart rates, blood pressure, and temperature are critical in emergency cases, "but in day-to-day life, the normalcy of those numbers is expected. It doesn't so much grant you a clean bill of health as indicate that you are not in acute danger."[40] Instead, Hamblin suggests, physicians hope that simple functional metrics may be able to replace measurements of the resting body. The intensity of the focus on body weight has only exacerbated the risks of eating disorders, body dysmorphias, anxiety and depression, social isolation, and many other issues that may be far more damaging to health than overweight or obesity. And those costs are not distributed evenly, with girls and women bearing the largest burden of the intense focus on weight. While functional tests, such as walking speed or a pushup test, are likely better screening tools than BMI, the history of standard weight tables suggests that it is very easy for social values to become deeply embedded in even the simplest of measures.[41] And while functional metrics may be better *measures* of nutrition and health than weight, they can just as easily (if not more so) become yet another source of competition or another burden that children must bear in the relentless quest for bodily conformity. Like weight, functional tests place responsibility on the individual to self-monitor and self-improve, providing simply one more way to create variable standards, and it is not hard to imagine how such standards may become gendered: would the pushup test involve "real" pushups or "girl" pushups?[42]

Notes

1. Clay Jones (@SBMPediatrics), Twitter post, January 9, 2019, 7:52 P.M. GMT, https://twitter.com/SBMPediatrics/status/1083089261145088003?s=03.
2. Clay Jones (@SBMPediatrics), Twitter post, January 9, 2019, 7:54 P.M. GMT, https://twitter.com/SBMPediatrics/status/1083089697046515713.

3. L. Emmett Holt, *Your Opportunity in the Schools* (Washington, D.C.: U.S. Bureau of Education, Health Education No. 9, 1922), 10, 12.

4. *Rules of the State Board of Health Relating to the Sanitary Care of Schools* (Madison: Wisconsin State Board of Health, 1920), 8. In 1925, the American Child Health Association (ACHA) surveyed eighty-six cities with populations between 40,000 and 70,000 people. Of those, 71 percent claimed weighing and measuring were part of the school health program, 56 percent reported that all schools had scales, and 80 percent weighed school children at least once a year. George T. Palmer et al., *A Health Survey of 86 Cities* (New York: American Child Health Association, 1925), 153.

5. On the history of weighing and measuring children to assess nutritional status and medico-scientific criticisms of the practice, see A. R. Ruis, "'Children with Half-Starved Bodies' and the Assessment of Malnutrition in the United States, 1890–1950," *Bulletin of the History of Medicine* 87, no. 3 (2013): 380–408.

6. Michel Foucault, *Technologies of the Self: A Seminar with Michel Foucault* (Cambridge: University of Massachusetts Press, 1988).

7. Jeffrey P. Brosco, "Weight Charts and Well Child Care: When the Pediatrician Became the Expert in Child Health," in *Formative Years: Children's Health in the United States, 1880–2000*, ed. Alexandra Minna Stern and Howard Markel (Ann Arbor: University of Michigan Press, 2004), 91–120.

8. Taliaferro Clark, "Nutrition in Schoolchildren," *Journal of the American Medical Association* 79, no. 7 (1922): 525.

9. Sydney A. Halpern, *American Pediatrics: The Social Dynamics of Professionalism, 1880–1980* (Berkeley: University of California Press, 1988); Richard A. Meckel, *Classrooms and Clinics: Urban Schools and the Protection and Promotion of Child Health, 1870–1930* (New Brunswick, NJ: Rutgers University Press, 2013); A. R. Ruis, "'Trois Empreintes d'Un Même Cachet': Toward a Historical Definition of Nutrition," in *Viral Networks: Connecting Digital Humanities and Medical History*, ed. E. Thomas Ewing and Katherine Randall (Blacksburg: VT Publishing, 2018), 179–212.

10. William R. P. Emerson, "The Class Method in the Dietetic and Hygienic Treatment of Delicate Children," *Pediatrics* 21 (1910): 626–27. For other descriptions of the nutrition class method, see William Henry Donnelly, "The Class Method of Treating Malnutrition in Children," *New York Medical Journal*, December 18, 1920, 973–75; William R. P. Emerson, *Nutrition Clinics and Classes: Their Organization and Conduct* (Boston, 1919); Susan Mathews, *Nutrition Class Helps* (Georgia State College of Agriculture, 1923); Lucy Oppen, "The Nutrition Class: An Opportunity for Preventive Work," *Hospital Social Service Quarterly* 1 (1919): 86–94; Frank Howard Richardson, *The Nutrition Class Idea: A Retrospect and a Prospect* (New York, 1921); Charles Hendee Smith, *The Nutrition Class* (New York: Child Health Organization, 1921).

11. Molly Ladd-Taylor, *Mother-Work: Women, Child Welfare, and the State, 1890–1930* (Urbana: University of Illinois Press, 1994); Richard A. Meckel, *Classrooms and Clinics: Urban Schools and the Protection and Promotion of Child Health, 1870–1930* (New Brunswick, NJ: Rutgers University Press, 2013); Naomi Rogers, "Vegetables on Parade: American Medicine and the Child Health Movement in the Jazz Age," in *Children's Health Issues in Historical Perspective*, ed. Cheryl Krasnick Warsh and Veronica Strong-Boag (Wilfrid Laurier University Press, 2005), 23–71; A. R. Ruis, *Eating to Learn, Learning to Eat: The Origins of School Lunch in the United States* (New Brunswick, NJ: Rutgers University Press, 2017); Elizabeth Toon, "Teaching Children about Health," in *Children and Youth in Sickness and Health: A Historical Handbook and*

Guide, ed. Janet Golden, Richard A. Meckel, and Heather Munro Prescott (New York: Greenwood, 2004), 85–105.

12. Alice H. Wood, "Nutrition Classes in the Chicago Schools," *Modern Medicine* 2, no. 5 (1920).

13. William R. P. Emerson, "Measured Feeding for Older Children," *Boston Medical & Surgical Journal* 170, no. 3 (1914): 81.

14. Lucy Oppen, *Teaching Health* (Washington, D.C.: U.S. Bureau of Education, Health Education No. 4, 1919), 3. See also Dorothy Hutchinson, *Suggestions for a Program for Health Teaching in the High School* (Washington, D.C.: U.S. Bureau of Education, Health Education No. 15, 1923), 2.

15. Advertisement for National Oats, *Ladies' Home Journal*, October 1919, 116.

16. For more on the "new" health education, see n. 11.

17. Ellen H. Richards, *Euthenics, the Science of Controllable Environment: A Plea for Better Living Conditions as a First Step toward Higher Human Efficiency* (Boston: Whitcomb & Barrows, 1910).

18. Mary Robert Baynham and Bertha K. Whipple, "A Nutrition Problem with Special Reference to Negro Children," *American Journal of Clinical Medicine*, August 1925, 309.

19. Richards, *Euthenics, the Science of Controllable Environment*, 4.

20. Rachel Louise Moran, *Governing Bodies: American Politics and the Shaping of the Modern Physique* (Philadelphia: University of Pennsylvania Press, 2018).

21. On lack of home control as a root cause of malnourishment, see Lydia J. Roberts, *Nutrition Work with Children* (Chicago: University of Chicago Press, 1927), 104.

22. Jean Lee Hunt, Buford J. Johnson, and Edith M. Lincoln, *Health Education and the Nutrition Class* (New York: New York City Bureau of Educational Experiments, 1921), 73. On Roosevelt's bodily transformation, see Gail Bederman, *Manliness and Civilization: A Cultural History of Gender and Race in the United States, 1880–1917* (University of Chicago Press, 1995).

23. Katharine A. Fisher, *The Lunch Hour at School* (Washington, D.C.: U.S. Bureau of Education, 1920), 28.

24. Alonzo Smith, Sadie S. Hobday, and E. Lucille Reid, "Health Service in a Negro District," *Journal of the National Medical Association* 22, no. 2 (1929): 68–74.

25. See, for example, Ellen M. Bartlett, "Building Up Underweight School Children: Malnourished Pupils in San Francisco Schools Show Improvement under New Program of Nutrition Work," *American Food Journal* 18, no. 5 (1923): 232; John C. Gebhart, *Malnutrition and School Feeding* (Washington, D.C.: U.S. Bureau of Education, 1921), 31–32; C. P. Knight, "Progress Report on Field Investigations in Child Hygiene in the State of Missouri to June 30, 1920," *Public Health Reports* 35, no. 53 (1920): 3152.

26. Lucy Oppen, *Wanted: Teachers to Enlist for Child Health Service* (Washington, D.C.: U.S. Bureau of Education, 1919), 4.

27. Taliaferro Clark, "Nutrition in Schoolchildren," *Journal of the American Medical Association* 79, no. 7 (1922): 519.

28. Clark, 524–25. See also Borden S. Veeder, *Preventive Pediatrics* (New York: D. Appleton & Co., 1926), 154.

29. Brosco, "Weight Charts and Well Child Care," 109–10.

30. Steven Shapin, "Why Was 'Custom a Second Nature' in Early Modern Medicine?" *Bulletin of the History of Medicine* 93, no. 1 (2019): 24.

31. Rima D. Apple, "Science Gendered: Nutrition in the United States, 1840–1940," *Clio Medica* 32 (1995): 129–54; Mary I. Barber, *History of the American Dietetic Association 1917–1959* (Philadelphia: J. B. Lippincott, 1959); Adelia M. Beeuwkes,

E. Neige Todhunter, and Emma Seifrit Weigley, eds., *Essays on History of Nutrition and Dietetics* (American Dietetic Association, 1967); Paul V. Betters, *The Bureau of Home Economics: Its History, Activities and Organization* (Washington, D.C.: Brookings Institution, 1930); Jo Anne Cassell, *Carry the Flame: The History of the American Dietetic Association* (American Dietetic Association, 1990); Julia Grant, "Modernizing Mothers: Home Economics and the Parent Education Movement, 1920–1945," in *Rethinking Home Economics: Women and the History of a Profession*, ed. Sarah Stage and Virginia B. Vincenti (New York: Cornell University Press, 1997), 55–74.

32. C. E. Turner, "Precision and Reliability of Underweight Measurement," *American Journal of Public Health* 19 (1929): 969–979, data on 970.

33. Henry P. Bowditch, *The Growth of Children: A Supplementary Investigation* (Boston: Rand, Aberg, & Co., 1879). On the difficulty of identifying hereditary and environmental contributions to body composition, see Franz Boaz, *Changes in Bodily Form of Descendants of Immigrants* (Washington, D.C.: Government Printing Office, 1910); C. B. Davenport, *Body Build: Its Development and Inheritance* (Washington, D.C.: Carnegie Institute of Washington, 1925).

34. Bird T. Baldwin, "The Use and Abuse of Weight-Height-Age Tables as Indexes of Health and Nutrition," *Journal of the American Medical Association* 82, no. 1 (1924): 1–4.

35. *Height and Weight as an Index of Nutrition* (New York: New York Nutrition Council, 1922), n.p. The application of aggregate data to individuals without having performed a regression analysis is a basic statistical fallacy (ecological fallacy). Anthropometrists had cautioned against commission of this fallacy as early as the mid-nineteenth century. See, for example, Benjamin Apthorp Gould, *Investigations in the Military and Anthropological Statistics of American Soldiers* (New York: Hurd & Houghton, 1869), 116; W. Townsend Porter, "On the Application to Individual School Children of the Mean Values Derived from Anthropological Measurements by the Generalizing Method," *Quarterly Publications of the American Statistical Association* 3 (1893): 576–87, esp. 579.

36. Turner, "Precision and Reliability of Underweight Measurement," 970.

37. Charles Hendee Smith, *The Nutrition Class* (New York: Child Health Organization, 1921), 9.

38. Raymond Franzen, *Physical Measures of Growth and Nutrition* (New York: American Child Health Association, 1929), 77.

39. Norman Jolliffe, "Nutritional Failures: Their Causes and Prevention," *Milbank Memorial Fund Quarterly* 20, no. 2 (1942): 117.

40. James Hamblin, "The Power of One Push-Up," *Atlantic*, June 27, 2019.

41. There is, of course, a very rich historiography on this issue. See, for example, Ian Hacking, *The Taming of Chance* (Cambridge: Cambridge University Press, 1990); Gerard Jorland, Annick Opinel, and George Weisz, eds., *Body Counts: Medical Quantification in Historical and Sociological Perspectives* (Montreal: McGill-Queen's University Press, 2005); Margaret A. Lowe, *Looking Good: College Women and Body Image, 1875–1930* (Baltimore: Johns Hopkins University Press, 2003); J. Rosser Matthews, *Quantification and the Quest for Medical Certainty* (Princeton, NJ: Princeton University Press, 1995).

42. Julia A. Valley and Kim C. Graber, "Gender-Biased Communication in Physical Education," *Journal of Teaching in Physical Education* 36, no. 4 (2017): 498–509.

Chapter 9

Competitive Youth Sports, Pediatricians, and Gender in the 1950s

Kathleen E. Bachynski

In 2018, retired National Football League (NFL) star Brett Favre told the *Daily Mail* that he would rather be remembered for ending youth tackle football than for his legendary Hall of Fame career. He supported legislation to prohibit tackle programs for young children, he said, explaining that "the body, the brain, the skull is not developed in your teens and single digits."[1] Favre was far from alone in his concern. In the wake of concussion lawsuits against the NFL and National Collegiate Athletic Association (NCAA), autopsies of former NFL players that revealed a degenerative neurological disease, and even a 2015 feature film on the subject starring actor Will Smith, a prominent national conversation developed over the risks of brain injuries in youth sports. Much of the discussion centered on American football, a sport played almost exclusively by boys. Advocates for youth football argued that the sport fostered a "brotherhood bond" and taught "toughness and aggressiveness."[2] Critics, on the other hand, emphasized the physical risks. "Tackle Can Wait," a campaign to promote flag football as a safer alternative, even likened tackling to smoking.[3]

Amid rising public awareness of concussion risks, in 2015, the American Academy of Pediatrics (AAP) issued a formal statement on the health effects of tackling in youth football. Despite acknowledging that eliminating tackling would likely reduce the incidence of concussions, severe injuries, catastrophic injuries, and overall injuries among child athletes, the AAP made no specific recommendation against football for children of any age.[4] Instead, the AAP's Council on Sports Medicine and Fitness indicated that athletes themselves must decide whether "the recreational benefits associated with proper tackling" outweighed the potential health risks. The AAP explained this decision by noting that removing tackling from football "would lead to a fundamental change in the way the game is played," something the council of pediatricians was not prepared to advise.[5] By 2015, competitive sports for children, particularly tackle football for boys, had become so entrenched in American society that even pediatricians charged with prioritizing children's health hesitated to counsel against a full-body collision sport.

In contrast, pediatricians were far more wary of organized youth sports when competitive programs for elementary and middle school–aged children took off in popularity after World War II. The mid-twentieth-century expansion of highly competitive sports was largely targeted at boys and was motivated in part by gendered beliefs about national defense needs and boys' inherent competitive drives. One national sports columnist defended "big league baseball in miniature" for boys aged eight to twelve by observing that "boys will be boys and they will compete in whatever they do."[6] Organizations such as Little League Baseball and Pop Warner Football featured corporate sponsorship, national broadcasts, national newspaper coverage, and heavy parental involvement.[7] They hosted regional, nationwide, and occasionally even international tournaments that often mimicked those of their adult counterparts. Notably, in 1957, President Eisenhower met that year's Little League world champions, a young team from Monterrey, Mexico, that had traveled to the United States to compete (see figure 9.1). The president described twelve-year-old pitcher and team captain Ángel Macias as "just like Mickey Mantle," the professional baseball legend.[8]

The potential effects of these trends in organized athletics on children's physical and emotional health troubled many doctors and educators. Pediatricians were foremost among the medical professionals who challenged the extension of highly competitive sports to young children in the 1950s. Focusing on the AAP's 1956 policy statement on competitive athletics, as well as AAP committee members' medical journal articles and statements in the popular press, this essay examines how gender influenced pediatricians' midcentury advice regarding competitive sports for young children. Beliefs about gender differences, puberty, and physical risk informed how pediatricians critiqued prevailing trends while simultaneously conceding the importance of competitive play for boys and girls in the Cold War era.

Sports for Future Warriors

After World War II, increasing prosperity, suburbanization, and public–private partnerships contributed to the expansion of youth sports programs.[9] Through initiatives such as Hale America and Operation Fitness USA, from the 1940s

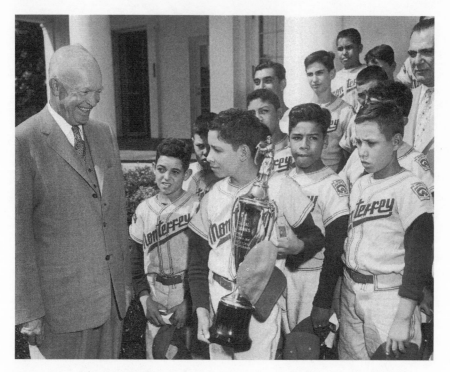

Figure 9.1. President Eisenhower meets the 1957 world champion Little League team from Monterrey, Mexico, at the White House. Team captain Ángel Macías holds the trophy. Courtesy of the National Archives, Dwight D. Eisenhower Presidential Library and Museum.

through the 1960s, the U.S. government partnered with "corporate, nonprofit, civic and religious organizations to advance the importance of physical fitness as both an individual and a patriotic necessity for men, women, and children."[10] But while a number of youth fitness programs included girls, competitive sports programs for preteens in both schools and external leagues were primarily for boys. For example, by 1954, the *Christian Science Monitor* reported that the previous year, 11,496 Little League Baseball teams were operating in forty-six states and estimated that 250,000 boys had played under the aegis of the Little League. No comparable program then existed for girls, prompting Barbara Ponticello of Newark, New Jersey, to write to Little League Baseball, "We're tired of being left out of everything. We want to play baseball like the boys." Little League Baseball would not officially admit girls until 1974.[11]

Several gendered anxieties, particularly concerns about juvenile delinquency and military preparedness, influenced the growth of competitive sports for boys. After World War II, American politicians, religious leaders, social scientists, physicians, law enforcement officials, and other prominent figures urged action to address the threat of juvenile delinquency.[12] They largely attributed the problem to boys, and especially to perceived failures in male socialization. This focus is evident, for example, in the title of American criminologist Albert K. Cohen's influential 1955 book, *Delinquent Boys: The Culture of the Gang.*[13] Moreover, doctors warned that failures in male socialization could begin early. Pediatrician Harry Bakwin emphasized that juvenile delinquents often began getting into trouble when they were as young as elementary school age. He contended that such boys were largely uncooperative, unconventional, and resistant to authority. "For amusements delinquent boys generally seek adventurous activities rather than competitive sports or games or quiet pursuits."[14] On this popular view, competitive sports not only were a normal boyhood pursuit but would also inculcate in boys the very qualities juvenile delinquents lacked, such as a cooperative attitude and respect for authority.

Concerns about men's physical fitness for selective service, particularly in the wake of World War II, also informed the expansion of competitive sports for boys. For example, in 1944, Commander Gene Tunney of the U.S. Navy Reserve called for a compulsory physical fitness program for youth after the war, contending that his military experience had influenced his perspective on "the essentiality of sports for the future warrior."[15] In 1948, Major General Maxwell Taylor, superintendent of the military academy at West Point, and G. Ott Romney, dean of the School of Physical Education and Athletics at West Virginia University, both urged an expanded physical education program as "essential to the well-being of our nation." Romney called for such a training program to begin in the first grade, with "competitive sports as its nucleus."[16] The reinstatement of the draft in 1950 due to the Korean War amplified such concerns about youth fitness.[17] Particularly given that only men were eligible to be drafted in military service, rhetoric of the period that connected soldiers and athletes nearly exclusively referred to boys and men.

Highly competitive sports programs for younger boys were also promoted as "feeder" systems for future high school or college play. For example, in his 1951 master's thesis on athletics in Tucson junior high schools, a University of Arizona graduate student described "a prominent member of the community" informing him that his local high school would soon begin to "reap the harvest" of the junior high school's intensive football program. "Upon questioning it was found that the junior high school boys played a seven game schedule of regulation football—traveling as far as 225 miles for one game."[18] In 1949, a junior high school principal decried widespread exploitation of grade school boys to produce winning high school teams alongside the proliferation of banquets, frequent trips, and "letters as large as the ones awarded high-school lettermen."[19] That same year, William P. Uhler of New Jersey's Department of Education highlighted some of the gender implications of these trends. He described a school where a high percentage of girls participated in intramural activities, but varsity sports programs were available only to boys. "Let us not forget that, of the 1,000 pupils, the development of the 940 not on the football squad is of far greater importance, though less spectacular, than the athletic success of the team."[20] By this view, the expansion of highly competitive sports programs exposed a minority of young boys to the harms of intensive athletics while depriving the rest of intramural athletic opportunities.

By 1949, the proliferation of highly competitive sports programs aimed at prepubescent boys prompted several national health and education organizations to form a joint committee to examine the issue. To address physiological factors related to athletic participation among children of elementary and junior high school age, the committee sent surveys to 424 physicians. They received 220 completed questionnaires, including 78 from pediatricians, the medical field with the highest response rate. The American Association for Health, Physical Education, and Recreation published the resulting report, *Desirable Athletic Competition for Children*, in 1952. The report recommended voluntary intramural activities for boys and girls in upper elementary grades and above but advised against interschool competition below ninth grade. In particular, the report warned that high-pressure elements such as tournaments, long seasons, or bowl games could make undue physical demands on both boys and girls.[21]

The report also included responses to a set of questions regarding psychological factors from psychiatrists, psychologists, pediatricians, and other experts in child growth and development. One question focused on gender differences: specifically, "do girls respond differently from boys of the same age level in similar athletic situations?" Of the fourteen experts who responded to this question, most indicated that there were no inherent differences or mentioned differences related to cultural expectations or "sex roles." For example, pediatrician Myron E. Wegman told the committee, "Girls do not ordinarily go in for the competitive sports involving bodily contact but when they do my observation has been that they play just as vigorously and with just as much feeling as the boys do." An educational psychologist described and dissented from a prevailing societal expectation that girls "give up" team sports and track after puberty.[22]

On the other hand, four respondents indicated that there were differences due to sex, claiming, for example, that "girls tend to be more expressive in their emotional outbursts." A physician emphasized that any activity that might harm "the girl's normal function as a mother should be discouraged." Overall, while the report made similar recommendations for athletic activities for young boys and girls, its survey responses recognized widespread cultural beliefs that then informed divergent athletic offerings for children according to gender. The view that puberty rendered competitive team sports inappropriate for girls was likely due, at least in part, to concerns that girls' future "normal" function as mothers should be prioritized. Furthermore, as another researcher highlighted, the "violent bodily contact of certain sports" was not considered "ladylike." Even the experts who disagreed with these perspectives acknowledged their cultural force. In focusing its recommendations on prepubescent children, the committee largely avoided the period of adolescence when gender distinctions in athletics were considered most relevant, but such beliefs are nonetheless evident in the report.[23]

In presenting the report to the public, committee chair Simon A. McNeely of the U.S. Office of Education told a reporter that the expansion of highly competitive sports to young children was doubtless done by people with "the best of intentions." He noted that businesses, civic clubs, and, in some cases, police departments sponsored the programs, the latter group with the goal of combatting juvenile delinquency. Despite these good intentions, McNeely and the committee advised that such highly competitive programs could be harmful to young children and advised occasional informal, intramural games instead. At the same time, McNeely felt compelled to add, "I'd like to have the idea emphasized that we're for sports and we're for competition. I don't want people thinking we're a bunch of fuddy-duddies." His comments reveal the challenging, and gendered, terrain the committee had to navigate in attempting to effectively advise against competitive sports programs, then expanding for young boys without coming across as overly cautious.[24]

Following the 1952 publication of *Desirable Athletic Competition for Children*, other medical and educational groups increasingly began to mention the topic, including the AAP's Committee on School Health. One of the AAP's oldest committees, the Committee on School Health, had been established in June 1931, just a year after the formation of the AAP. The committee had initially focused on inspecting schoolchildren for infectious diseases and physical disabilities that could impede their education but would soon address many other topics related to school health.[25] In a 1954 medical journal report, the Committee on School Health briefly described health concerns related to youth athletics, concluding with the committee's belief that "an organized study is necessary to determine the effects of competitive athletics on the health of school age children."[26]

In addition, George Maksim, a member of the AAP's Committee on School Health, penned a 1953 article on youth sports in the *National Parent-Teacher Magazine* in which he warned against parents expecting of children "a maturity far beyond what the normal processes of nature have accomplished." Maksim claimed that boys younger than thirteen were five to ten times more likely to get injured playing tackle football than older teenagers, while brain damage could result from boxing "and effects may be permanent." He counseled against body contact sports and advised instead a more universal program of athletics for both genders to involve children of all physical abilities. "All boys and girls in every community should have an outlet for their energies and their competitive instincts in the form of a properly organized, properly supervised sports program. . . . Even the handicapped child can serve as a team manager, scorekeeper, or member of the band." Maksim recommended several sports he considered suitable for both boys and girls, such as track and field events, volleyball, tennis, and rope jumping.[27]

But the AAP much more directly engaged with the topic of athletic competition for young children after Dwight D. Eisenhower weighed in on the topic with the power of the presidency. A 1954 study finding that American schoolchildren had fared poorly on a measure of muscular fitness as compared to European children helped prompt Eisenhower's concern.[28] In July 1955, Eisenhower invited the authors of the study to speak at a White House luncheon, where he expressed alarm over the large proportion of youths rejected from military service for physical reasons.[29] In addition to enhancing children's physical fitness, Eisenhower also told the assembled sports leaders and other guests that more American youngsters should be encouraged to play competitive sports as one good way to fight juvenile delinquency.[30]

Eisenhower's pronouncements troubled pediatricians concerned about the health effects of intense sports programs for children. At the closing session of the AAP's annual meeting later that year, pediatricians John Reichert and George Maksim urged "a reinterpretation of President Eisenhower's July 11 call for more emphasis on competitive sports." The doctors diplomatically emphasized that they had no criticism of the president; rather, they feared a misinterpretation of his statement might result in too much stress placed on the competitive side of sports for children. Reichert issued a statement on behalf of the AAP's Committee on School Health, recognizing the need for regular exercise for children that should be provided through "a positive program of universal participation in a wide variety of sports and play activities." But the committee ruled out body contact sports, specifically boxing and football, for young children.[31]

The following week, Reichert and Maksim both attended the fifth National Conference on Physicians and Schools in Highland Park, Illinois. The American Medical Association and its Bureau of Health Education sponsored the conference, comprising doctors, public health officials, and educators. Maksim chaired a discussion on youth athletics that advocated for different approaches to sports for children younger than age twelve as compared to older children. Among older children, the group advised that athletics should be "on an intramural basis in the junior high schools and for girls in the senior high schools."[32]

In the wake of Eisenhower's call for more competitive sports among youth, then, pediatricians at these professional conferences instead advocated for fostering universal participation and avoiding high-stress competition among young children. For adolescents, they advised intramural sports for girls through high school but implied that interscholastic athletic competitions for high school–age boys were acceptable. These recommendations indicated that similar play activities could be offered for prepubescent children of both genders but that intense competition was not appropriate for young children. Meanwhile, the belief that going through puberty for boys might prepare them to engage in interscholastic sports, but that puberty did not have the same protective effect on girls, also informed the pediatricians' analysis.

To Play for the Fun of Playing

These attitudes toward gender shaped the AAP's next effort to address the issue by developing more formal guidelines on competitive youth sports. Eight male pediatricians from the AAP's Committee on School Health took up the task. Chaired by John Reichert, the group also included George Maksim as well as future AAP president George B. Logan. Reichert, born in 1896 and the son of a physician, had devoted his medical career to school health. The mayor of Chicago had appointed him to serve on the Chicago Board of Education, and in addition to the AAP's group, he also chaired school health committees of the Illinois Medical Society and the Chicago Pediatric Society.[33]

In 1956, *Pediatrics* published the committee's policy statement, focusing on children aged twelve and younger. The authors explained that amid controversy over competitive youth athletics, educators, community leaders, and especially parents were turning to doctors for guidance. The AAP committee intended their guidelines "to aid physicians in this advisory role" on youth sports. They analyzed the subject according to the factors of age, sex, competition, athletics, programs, physical aspects, emotional aspects, and leadership before concluding with a set of twelve recommendations. Beliefs about gender influenced how the AAP committee defined competition for children, its concerns about the risks of high-pressure sports, and the activities it recommended for boys and girls.[34]

The policy statement opened by acknowledging that while there were differences of opinion over the age at which particular activities should be introduced and how competitive they should be, "it is generally agreed that athletic programs for children of all ages are a necessary part of their education and recreation." The committee elaborated on this theme under the "competition" heading, explaining that competition could be defined as "as an attempt to surpass previous accomplishment singly or collectively." On this view, "vying with one another is not only part of our society but, as defined here, it is an inherent part of the growing, developing child." Children's inherent competitive drives needed to be guided so that competition and cooperation would be "properly balanced." But a primary emphasis on winning, or teachers or parents placing emotional pressures on children, would render athletic programs highly competitive and undesirable.[35]

The committee thus conceded the importance of competition for growing children while seeking to reframe the notion of healthy competition away from a focus on winning. By characterizing competition as a striving to improve one's own or collective performance, rather than to defeat an opponent, the committee was offering a framework for youth athletics that was consistent with President Eisenhower's call for increased competition without sanctioning high-pressure youth sports. Given that most organized competitive sports leagues were then designed for boys, the committee was also providing a more gender-neutral understanding of healthy play and athletic competition for young children.

Several concerns about physical and emotional development informed the committee's wariness of high-pressure athletics for young girls and boys. The AAP highlighted the potential effects of "greatly ballyhooed interscholastic or interleague competition" on physical maturation processes such as bone, joint, and muscle development, as well as the potential for chronic fatigue to interfere with healthy child growth. The committee was particularly worried about children aged twelve and under "because the growing ends of their long bones have not yet calcified, and because they do not possess the protection of adult musculature." The report emphasized that boys and girls were not "little men" or "little women" but children who would grow up "in Nature's own way and time." This phrasing suggested that competitive athletics were detrimental because they were unnatural for young children of both genders.[36]

The AAP report reiterated pediatricians' concerns over the effect of competitive sports on children's growth plates despite skepticism from coaches and sports administrators who doubted such risks existed in team sports, let alone interfered with the natural growth of the boys who participated in them. For example, in 1953, Eugene Nixon, a former Pomona College football coach, argued that most physicians made too much of possible injuries to the epiphyses, the end part of long bones where growth took place. "I'll be hornswoggled if in a half century of football I have encountered a boy or man who showed evidence of having been injured in the epiphyses," he wrote in the *Los Angeles Times*. Concluding with a message to his grandson interested in playing football, Nixon wrote, "Good luck to you and may you have seven or eight years of glorious football—and the heck with the epiphyses." While Nixon may have been usually vocal in his skepticism of medical advice, his commentary illustrates a pronounced divergence between pediatricians and sports coaches on the physiological effects of collision sports like football on child growth.[37]

The AAP committee was also positioning itself in opposition to claims that competitive sports, or even injuries sustained while playing competitive sports, could actively enhance normal childhood development. For example, Creighton Hale, a physiologist who would join Little League Baseball as its director of research in 1955, contended that there was an important distinction to be made between physical injury versus physiological harm. "In fact, a broken bone, as many know, may mend to be a stronger bone than it was before it was broken."[38] On this view, an injury was not only harmless but might ultimately strengthen the biological growth process.

Beliefs that exposure to danger and physical injury could foster "virile characteristics" and accelerate growth were gendered, often employed by coaches and administrators who advocated for competitive team sports for boys younger than high school age.[39] Improving boys' physical fitness was widely interpreted as increasing their muscular strength, growth, and toughness. Some researchers attributed the desire to "bulk up" to the boys themselves. For example, in 1947, the Denver Public Schools conducted an extensive survey of students' health interests. The report found that seventh-grade boys were most interested "to learn how to build muscles." By contrast, the committee reported that seventh-grade girls, "most of whom are in the early-adolescent period of growth, are primarily interested in being personally attractive."[40] A 1961 textbook on health education coedited by John Reichert noted that these findings were undoubtedly "an outgrowth of the expectations of family and peer culture."[41] Such cultural expectations regarding the desirability of muscle growth according to gender influenced the development of competitive athletic programs for boys but not for girls.

Those who opposed the expansion of highly competitive sports for boys, then, often cast doubt on the value of focusing on muscular growth. For example, one mother who wrote the *Chicago Daily Tribune* to decry this trend contended that due to the influence of athletic associations, American boys, "our future leaders, are grown into big hunks of meat."[42] By warning that competitive athletics for young children could interfere with natural growth, the AAP committee thus also implicitly challenged a prevailing view that organized sports would successfully transform boys into men. The AAP report suggested that competitive sports for young children might cause physical injury and "insidious interference with optimal body functions" that could result in both short-term and long-term harm, rather than fostering strength and body development.[43]

Although in practice, the AAP's concerns about the impact of competitive sports on physiological development most strongly challenged expanding athletic programs for boys, the committee expressed a heightened worry for girls. "The problems of growth and development are even more evident among girls, as some begin normally to mature before the age of 12 years." On this view, girls were particularly vulnerable to the risks of an overemphasis on intense athletic participation, leading the committee to opine that "fortunately, in most communities highly organized competitive sports are not available for girls." At the same time, the AAP decried the lack of any sports program for girls in most communities, which implied "that girls are being encouraged to be spectators only." Consequently, while agreeing with popular beliefs that young girls were especially susceptible to the dangers of competitive sports, the AAP objected to the common practice of excluding girls from active athletic participation and relegating them to the sidelines.[44]

By objecting to muscle testing as a marker of fitness, the AAP further challenged a gendered emphasis on muscular strength as a measure of child health. In so doing, the AAP committee did not directly refer to Eisenhower's speech but instead alluded to the study of muscular fitness in American versus European children that had prompted the president's concern. The study had "scared the nation," as one high school physical education director put it, and had made the Kraus-Weber test for muscular fitness "an educational 'hot potato.'"[45] Although the test was designed for both boys and girls, its focus on muscular strength also spurred a variety of commentary that primarily characterized the American youth in need of strengthening as boys. For example, in a 1956 article titled "Let's Beef Up Our Kids," one columnist praised a businessman who had enlisted the help of male sports champions to write "a physical-conditioning course designed to enable any kid to develop his body and learn self-defense." A boy seeking to develop his body by "beefing up" was the imagined audience for such courses, and the expansion of team sports associated with increased muscular strength similarly focused on boys.[46]

In this context, the AAP committee's objections to relying on the strength or flexibility of specific muscles to assess child health was consistent with its more gender-neutral interpretation of avoiding intense competition or using muscle measurements to mark physical well-being. The AAP report flatly stated that comparing the results of muscle testing in groups of children of different nationalities "is not a valid estimate of physical fitness or whether they are 'healthy' school children." Instead, the AAP advised athletic programs for both boys and girls that were "appropriate to the individual differences in children's capacities."[47]

The committee observed that few published statements had addressed athletics for girls, who represented about half of the elementary school population. "A proper program of games and sports is equally essential for girls and boys. . . . Sports programs which include calisthenics, folk dancing, kickball, baseball, swimming, skating, tennis, golf, archery and similar activities should be encouraged for both sexes." By recommending a broad list of activities for both boys and girls, the AAP promoted a vision of physical fitness programs "in which children of both sexes with varying abilities have an opportunity and are encouraged to participate freely." The AAP highlighted that all children would benefit from active participation in recreation and regular exercise. Moreover, the AAP advised that the overarching goal of youth athletics should include helping children "learn to play for the fun of playing" and that elementary school–level activities could include such nonathletic options as nature study, games, and hiking.[48]

On several important levels, then, the AAP's recommendations challenged prevailing attitudes that limited girls' athletic participation in the 1950s. Nearly two decades before the passage of Title IX increased girls' access to athletic programs and before Little League Baseball's decision to admit girls, the AAP was advising that girls could participate in recreational team sports such as kickball and baseball. The AAP also recommended a focus on more gender-neutral objectives for youth athletic programs in the context of widespread beliefs that highly competitive sports could "beef up" boys, prepare them to meet national defense needs, enhance their future athletic success in high school varsity programs, and prevent juvenile delinquency. On the other hand, the AAP reinforced other popular beliefs about gender differences, notably advising that "the difference in interests of boys and girls at various ages should be considered in planning programs," and echoing widely held concerns that girls were especially vulnerable to the risks of competition.[49]

Allowing a Boy to Take Part

In the years following the AAP's 1956 policy recommendations on competitive athletics, at least three of the statement's coauthors—George B. Logan, George Maksim, and John Reichert—continued to address the issue in medical journals and in interviews with news outlets. In 1957, Reichert penned an article titled "A Pediatrician's View of Competitive Sports before the Teens" for *Today's Health*. This publication of the American Medical Association was commonly left for patients to read in doctors' waiting rooms and often represented "the mainstream medical consensus on a wide variety of topics."[50] The article conveyed many of the same messages as the AAP's 1956 guidelines but included even more explicit critiques of competitive sports for boys. For example, Reichert warned that young boys were concealing injuries due to fears that "they would be accused of being sissies by their coaches or fellow players." Such medical advice countered the view expressed by political leaders and sports administrators that competitive body-contact sports benefited young boys by "toughening" them up.[51] In particular, it challenged the notion that boys ought to play sports in order to avoid "sissy" tendencies, a sexist term then widely used to characterize boys and men perceived as effeminate or homosexual. Instead, Reichert suggested that this cultural motivation to play through injuries was in fact harming boys' health.[52]

At the American Medical Association's 1958 annual meeting, both Logan and Maksim read papers on the topic of desirable athletic competition for children, which were subsequently published in separate issues of *JAMA*. Maksim's paper emphasized that "competition is part of our American way of life," but that programs for young children "should not include contact sports," again advocating for other forms of competition for both young boys and girls.[53] Similarly, Maksim told *Sports Illustrated* in a 1957 article on Little League Baseball, "Competition is part of the growing child that should be recognized, accepted and directed."[54] Particularly given the Cold War context in which competition was distinguished from Soviet communism as a key feature of the "American way of life," Maksim seems to have been particularly careful to endorse competition as an essential element of American childhood. Yet Maksim emphasized that age-appropriate competition did not need to include what he saw as undue pressure and commercialism in many highly organized team sports programs for boys.

Meanwhile, Logan focused on the importance of medical supervision, notably to examine boys to evaluate whether a prospective athlete could "hold his own in the proposed sport." Logan acknowledged that "no accurate test or measure is available for this purpose" but contended that physicians could nonetheless make a rough determination. For example, he advised that the development of pubic hair was often a helpful marker when evaluating high school boys. Logan's advice regarding preparticipation physicals largely framed the issue as being one of examining boys to determine whether they were sufficiently mature to play contact sports. For males, going through puberty was considered a sign of increased preparedness for engaging in contact sports. Logan also more strongly highlighted the emotional benefits of contact sports, particularly for older boys, as compared to the potential physical risks. "A fractured bone may leave less of a scar than a personality frustrated by parental timidity over allowing a boy to take part in a contact sport."[55] Logan's perspective more strongly identified contact sports with competition than previous statements from members of the AAP's Committee on School Health. It is no coincidence, then, that Logan also placed a greater emphasis on sports for boys.

In the final paragraph of the article's main section, before concluding with a reflection on physicians' professional responsibilities, Logan acknowledged that most articles on the topic concerned boys alone. But girls also needed medical supervision for athletic participation, he observed, though "customarily their sport activities are less strenuous and less intensively competitive than boys' sports, and they seldom engage in body contact sports." In contrast to the 1956 AAP guidelines, which prioritized activities for both boys and girls up to age twelve, Logan's 1959 *JAMA* article largely focused on medical supervision to make sports safe for boys as they matured, with girls' athletic involvement appearing more as an afterthought.[56]

The variations in these three pediatricians' advice were due in part to the extent to which they concurred with cultural narratives about competitive sports benefiting boys by toughening them up. Notably, Reichert highlighted boys' fears of being dubbed a "sissy" as harmful and exacerbating injuries, whereas Logan warned that "parental timidity" might frustrate boys' emotional and physical needs for competition by keeping them away from contact sports. As late as 1966, the AAP's Committee on School Health continued to recommend nonvarsity athletics as substitutes for intense interscholastic competition, advising that intramural programs were "one of the best means of allowing youngsters to develop wholesome attitudes about physical activity" and could account for "individual needs, differences, and interests."[57]

But by the 1960s, the perspective of sports medicine doctors who voiced support for competitive athletics, particularly for boys, was increasingly dominant. Pop Warner and Little League programs continued to expand, drawing hundreds of thousands of young male participants.[58] "Boys of all ages but especially pre-adolescents and adolescents dislike prolonged rest and restriction from action," explained the *Journal of Sports Medicine and Physical Fitness* in 1966.[59] The belief that youth sports served as an outlet for masculine energies and as a social inoculation against potential "sissy" tendencies largely overwhelmed pediatricians' efforts in the 1950s to encourage an intramural, universal athletic program for young children of both genders. The implications would be profound for American understandings of the risks and benefits of youth sports throughout the remainder of the twentieth century.

The Gendered Expansion of Competitive Youth Sports

Despite research documenting higher risks of injuries in contact and collision sports than lower contact alternatives, sports medicine doctors, coaches, and administrators continued to insist that the hazards were small in comparison to the advantages. As one orthopedic surgeon told the *Boston Globe* in 1972, "There is integration of body functions, cooperation with others, breakdown of social and economic barriers just to name a few of the kinds of benefits organized athletics can offer a boy."[60] Competitive sports leagues for elementary and middle school–aged boys proliferated and increasingly served as feeder systems for future high school and college play.[61] Schools and private leagues alike promoted athletic programs based on the view that competitive sports provided specific physical and emotional benefits to boys that other activities could not.

Moreover, gendered understandings of the advantages of contact sports shaped the expansion of athletic programs to women and girls following the passage of Title IX in 1972. In 1975, five pediatricians the AAP's Committee on Pediatric Aspects of Physical Fitness, Recreation and Sports published a commentary on girls' participation in sports. Alluding to Title IX, the committee opened by noting that "until recently, girls and women have been deprived of their rightful share in physical recreation and sports" and advised equal access for athletes of both genders to competent medical care, quality equipment, coaching, and playing facilities. Consistent with the AAP's recommendations in the 1950s, the committee advised that there was "no reason to separate prepubescent children by sex in sports." While older girls might compete against girls in any sport, however, the AAP warned that "postpubescent girls should not participate against boys in heavy collision sports because of the grave risk of serious injury due to their lesser muscle mass per unit of body weight." The

AAP concluded that investing in programs specifically for girls would yield greater benefits than focusing on "the exceptional female athlete" who might seek to participate in athletics on boys' teams.[62]

The high value placed upon competitive sports associated with physical strength and aggression influenced prevailing beliefs that athletic programs needed to remain gender segregated. On this view, equal opportunity for women and girls demanded a "separate but equal" approach to sports and fitness. As professor of kinesiology and sport history Joan Hult explained in 1973, "In at least two very important attributes for skilled performance—muscular strength and power—there is a definite difference between male and female. All the training and conditioning in the world cannot erase that truth."[63] The gendered benefits associated with competitive sports, such as fostering toughness and leadership skills, further informed the development of programs for women and girls. "Anything athletics can do for men, it can do for women in terms of developing leadership, making decisions, improving organization and shooting for goals," Sandra Scott, the associate director of the New York State Public High School Association, told the *New York Times*.[64] In 1979, the *Boston Globe* explained that as women increasingly joined the labor force, having experience playing sports became even more important. As management consultant Betty Harragan observed, "Once you work for pay, you are involved in a structure whose rules are modeled on competitive team sports."[65] On this view, by increasing their access to competitive team sports, Title IX would also enable girls and women to succeed in workplaces historically dominated by men.

Because the social benefits attributed to competitive sports remained gendered, so, too, did the justifications for the physical risks. In the 1980s and early 1990s, the growing privatization and commercialization of youth sports contributed to increasingly competitive programs as well as sports specialization at younger ages.[66] In 1991, two sports medicine physicians highlighted increasing patterns of injury due to these trends. They warned that children were particularly vulnerable to overuse injuries from repetitive training and should not be pressured into the rigors of competitive activity.[67] At the same time, doctors became increasingly reluctant to recommend against youth participation in team competition, even in collision sports. Although the AAP had formally recommended against body contact sports for boys and girls under twelve in the 1950s, by the twenty-first century, the AAP's Council on Sports Medicine and Fitness advised no limits on when children might begin to tackle one another.[68] In 2016, the AAP recommended against early specialization in sports that could lead to overuse injuries and burnout, noting that "unfortunately 70% of children drop out of organized sports by 13 years of age." The statement assumed that participation in organized sports was desirable for young children but recommended that they play multiple sports until puberty, so that injuries and burnout from a single sport would not hinder their future participation.[69]

Gendered understandings of the recreational benefits of full-body contact sports, in conjunction with the growing prominence of sports medicine, influenced the shift in the AAP's stance. Pediatricians concerned about the health risks were largely unable to rein in the mid-twentieth-century expansion of highly competitive sports for boys. Over time, the AAP increasingly adopted the gendered values that drove that expansion and influenced the extension of organized competitive sports to girls. Consequently, pediatric advice primarily focused on enhancing medical supervision of contact and collision sports instead of recommending lower-risk activities for young children.[70] Rather than the gender-neutral, low-pressure forms of recreation the AAP had advocated at the mid-twentieth century for prepubescent children, Americans largely embraced highly competitive, specialized, gender-segregated youth sports programs. Beliefs about gender, competition, and risk continue to inform medical advice about whether and how girls and boys should compete on fields, courts, and rinks across the United States.

Notes

1. Alex Raskin, "NFL Legend Brett Favre Would Rather Be Remembered for Ending Youth Tackle Football Than His Hall of Fame Career If It Means Saving Kids from Head Trauma He Endured for Decades," *Daily Mail*, June 20, 2018, https://www.dailymail.co.uk/news/article-5866131/Brett-Favre-remembered-ENDING-youth-tackle-football-Hall-Fame-career.html (accessed January 25, 2020).

2. Vin Sehgal, "7 Reasons in Favor of Kids Playing Tackle Football," *USA Football*, June 10, 2016, https://blogs.usafootball.com/blog/1374/7-reasons-in-favor-of-kids-playing-tackle-football (accessed January 26, 2020).

3. "Concussion PSA Compares Youth Football Dangers to Smoking," *NBC News*, October 10, 2019, https://www.nbcnews.com/news/us-news/concussion-psa-compares-youth-football-dangers-smoking-n1064581 (accessed January 25, 2020).

4. Kathleen E. Bachynski, "Tolerable Risks? Physicians and Youth Tackle Football," *New England Journal of Medicine* 374 (2016): 405–7.

5. American Academy of Pediatrics Committee on Sports Medicine and Fitness, "Tackling in Youth Football," *Pediatrics* 136, no. 5 (2015): e1419–30.

6. Arthur Daley, "Sports of the Times: In Mild Rebuttal," *New York Times*, September 12, 1952.

7. Jack W. Berryman, "From the Cradle to the Playing Field: America's Emphasis on Highly Organized Competitive Sports for Preadolescent Boys," *Journal of Sport History* 2 (1976): 112–31; Michael H. Carriere, "'A Diamond Is a Boy's Best Friend': The Rise of Little League Baseball, 1939–1964," *Journal of Sport History* 32, no. 3 (2005): 351–78.

8. "Little League Champions Meet and Cheer 'Senor Presidente,'" *New York Times*, August 28, 1957.

9. Carriere, "A Diamond Is a Boy's Best Friend," Kathleen Bachynski, *No Game for Boys to Play: The History of Youth Tackle Football and the Origins of a Public Health Crisis* (Chapel Hill: University of North Carolina Press, 2019).

10. Jaime Schultz, *Qualifying Times: Points of Change in U.S. Women's Sport* (Urbana: University of Illinois Press, 2014), 85.

11. Emilie Tavel, "Little League: Good or Bad?" *Christian Science Monitor*, August 25, 1954; Arthur Daley, "The Little League Is Big Time," *New York Times*, May 25, 1952; Douglas E. Abrams, "The Twelve-Year-Old Girl's Lawsuit That Changed America: The Continuing Impact of Now v. Little League Baseball, Inc. at 40," *Virginia Journal of Social Policy and the Law* 20 (2012): 241–69.

12. James Gilbert, *A Cycle of Outrage: America's Reaction to the Juvenile Delinquent in the 1950s* (Oxford: Oxford University Press, 1986).

13. Albert K. Cohen, *Delinquent Boys: The Culture of the Gang* (Glencoe, IL: Free Press, 1955).

14. Harry Bakwin, "Causes of Juvenile Delinquency," *AMA American Journal of Diseases of Children* 89, no. 3 (1955): 368–73.

15. "Tunney Advocates Youth Fitness after World War," *Daily Boston Globe*, October 19, 1944.

16. Lucy Freeman, "Truman Board Hit on Athletics Lack," *New York Times*, April 9, 1948.

17. Howard Rusk, "How Healthy Is America's Youth?" *New York Times*, May 6, 1951.

18. George Ellison McConnell, "An Evaluation of the Athletic Program in the Junior High Schools of Tucson, Arizona" (Master's Thesis, University of Arizona, 1951), 13.

19. A. H. Lauchner, "Boys in Grades Exploited for High School Teams," *The Clearing House* 24, no. 3 (1949): 133.

20. William P. Uhler, "So This Is Education," *Journal of the American Association for Health, Physical Education, and Recreation* 20, no. 10 (1949): 644, 691.

21. Joint Committee on Athletic Competition for Children of Elementary and Junior High School Age, *Desirable Athletic Competition for Children: Joint Committee Report* (Washington, D.C.: AAHPER, 1952).

22. Joint Committee, *Desirable Athletic Competition*, 20.

23. Joint Committee, *Desirable Athletic Competition*, 20.

24. Arthur Edson, "Educators Tee Off on Kids' Leagues," *Washington Post*, December 19, 1952. See also Bachynski, *No Game for Boys to Play*.

25. Marshall Pease, *American Academy of Pediatrics: June 1930 to June 1951* (Evanston, IL: American Academy of Pediatrics, 1952). In a 1954 report, the Committee on School Health acknowledged that the term "school health" perplexed many physicians and could be better defined as a "health program for school age children." AAP Committee on School Health, "Report of the Committee on School Health: School Health Policies," *Pediatrics* 13, no. 1 (1954): 74–82.

26. AAP Committee on School Health, "Report of the Committee on School Health."

27. George Maksim, "A Pediatrician's Views on Sports for Children," *National Parent-Teacher* 48, no. 4 (1953): 20–22.

28. Hans Kraus and Bonnie Prudden, "Minimum Muscular Fitness Tests in School Children," *Research Quarterly* 5, no. 2 (1954), 178–98; Bachynski, *No Game for Boys to Play*.

29. Jack Walsh, "Condition of Youth Alarms Eisenhower," *Washington Post and Times Herald*, July 12, 1955.

30. "Ike Calls for Increase in Competitive Sports," *Daily Boston Globe,* July 12, 1955; "President Invites 32 Sports Leaders," *New York Times,* July 10, 1955.

31. "Sport Rivalry for Children Is Criticized," *Chicago Daily Tribune,* October 7, 1955.

32. "School Conference on Health Problems," *Journal of the American Medical Association* 159, no. 11 (1955): 1126–28.

33. Herman F. Meyer, "John Lester Reichert, 1896–1964," *Proceedings of the Institute of Medicine of Chicago* 25 (1965): 236–37.

34. AAP Committee on School Health, "Competitive Athletics: A Statement of Policy," *Pediatrics* 18 (1956): 672–76.

35. AAP Committee on School Health, "Competitive Athletics," 673.

36. AAP Committee on School Health, "Competitive Athletics," 673.

37. Eugene Nixon, "Hang the Epiphyses: Nixon Gives Young Teen-Agers Green Light to Play Football," *Los Angeles Times*, September 13, 1953.

38. "Athletic Competition for Children?" *Athletic Journal* 34, no. 5 (1954): 18, 20, 55.

39. Charles Mather, "A Brief for Junior High School Football," *Scholastic Coach* 21, no. 2 (April 1952): 32–36.

40. Denver Public Schools, *Health Interests of Children* (Denver, CO: Denver Public Schools, 1947).

41. Bernice R. Moss, Warren H. Southworth, and John L. Reichert, eds., *Health Education: A Guide for Teachers and a Text for Teacher Education*, 5th ed. (Chicago: National Educational Association of the United States, 1961), 175.

42. Edith Marsh, "Muscle Factories," *Chicago Daily Tribune*, February 14, 1950.

43. AAP Committee on School Health, "Competitive Athletics," 673.

44. AAP Committee on School Health, "Competitive Athletics," 672.

45. Ed Comerford, "How Fit Is American Youth?" *Newsday*, March 1, 1957.

46. Hal Boyle, "The Boyle-ing Point: Let's Beef Up Our Kids," *Newsday*, May 9, 1956.

47. AAP Committee on School Health, "Competitive Athletics," 674.

48. AAP Committee on School Health, "Competitive Athletics," 674.

49. AAP Committee on School Health, "Competitive Athletics," 672.

50. Elizabeth Siegel Watkins, *The Estrogen Elixir: A History of Hormone Replacement Therapy in America* (Baltimore: Johns Hopkins University Press, 2007), 71.

51. John L. Reichert, "A Pediatrician's View of Competitive Sports before the Teens," *Today's Health* 35 (1957): 28–31.

52. Thomas Wendelboe, "A Cure for the Common Sissy: Masculine Health Consumption in the Cold War Era" (MA Thesis, University of New Brunswick, 2010).

53. George Maksim, "Desirable Athletics for Children," *JAMA* 168, no. 11 (1958): 1431–33.

54. Kenneth Rudeen, "The Verdict," *SI*, August 26, 1957.

55. George B. Logan, "Essential Medical Supervision in Athletics for Children," *JAMA* 169, no. 8 (1959): 786–88.

56. Logan, 788.

57. AAP Committee on School Health, *Report of the Committee on School Health of the American Academy of Pediatrics* (Evanston, IL: American Academy of Pediatrics, 1966), 72.

58. Kathleen E. Bachynski; "'The Duty of Their Elders'—Doctors, Coaches, and the Framing of Youth Football's Health Risks, 1950s–1960s," *Journal of the History of Medicine and Allied Sciences* 74, no. 2 (2019): 167–91.

59. Augustin Castellanos and Pedro Greer, "Tackle Football in Pre–High School Children," *Journal of Sports Medicine and Physical Fitness* 6, no. 3 (1966): 187–90.

60. Carl Cobb, "Football, Hockey Top Schoolboy Injuries," *Boston Globe*, November 18, 1972.
61. Bachynski, *No Game for Boys to Play*.
62. Melvin L. Thornton, Gloria D. Eng, Jon H. Kennell, et al., "Participation in Sports by Girls," *Pediatrics* 55 (1975): 563.
63. Joan Hult, "Girls' and Women's Sports," *Journal of Health, Physical Education and Recreation* 44, no. 6 (1973): 57–58.
64. Robert Hanley, "Girls Now Gaining Fast on Boys in Team Athletics in High School," *New York Times*, April 5, 1984.
65. Signe Hammer, "My Daughter, the Football Star," *Boston Globe*, August 5, 1979.
66. Jay Coakley, "The 'Logic' of Specialization," *Journal of Physical Education, Recreation & Dance* 81, no. 8 (2010): 16–18, 25.
67. Lyle J. Micheli and J. D. Klein, "Sports Injuries in Children and Adolescents," *British Journal of Sports Medicine* 25, no. 1 (1991): 6–9.
68. American Academy of Pediatrics Committee on Sports Medicine and Fitness, "Tackling in Youth Football."
69. Joel S. Brenner, "Sports Specialization and Intensive Training in Young Athletes," *Pediatrics* 138, no. 3 (2016): e1–e8.
70. Bachynski, "Tolerable Risks?"

Chapter 10

Gender and the "New" Puberty

Heather Munro Prescott

The belief that children are entering puberty at younger ages today than they did in the past has been a topic of considerable debate in the pediatric literature and popular media over the past two decades. In 1997, a research group at the University of North Carolina School of Public Health, led by Marcia Herman-Giddens, released a study of 17,000 girls from around the country indicating that the average age of onset of puberty had declined by six months to one year since the mid-twentieth century. The study found notable racial differences in pubertal timing as well: African American girls started puberty, as indicated by the appearance of breast buds and pubic hair, at an average of one year earlier than white girls.[1] Four years later, the same research team published an article stating that boys were also entering puberty at earlier ages than in the past and that the change was most remarkable among African American boys.[2] Although some pediatric researchers questioned the reliability of these studies, others contended—and still do—that children in the modern industrialized world are experiencing a "new puberty" that begins well before the teenage years.[3]

When these findings first came out, they led to an outpouring of alarmist reports in the popular press about the social and medical implications of children who started puberty in elementary school. These articles reveal cultural preoccupations about gender, race, and sexuality as they relate to children's bodies. For example, a photo-essay published in 2000 in the *New York Times Magazine* featured an interview with Herman-Giddens, who speculated on the various causes—sexual images in the media, rising rates of obesity, growth hormones in milk—that could be causing accelerated maturation.[4] Sociologist Celia

Roberts observes that these stories have created a new sense of "crisis" around puberty, one that focuses overwhelmingly on female sexual development.[5]

Yet this is not the first time that Americans have used the developing bodies of children and adolescents as a trope for broader social and cultural anxieties. As the historian Paula Fass has observed, adults have often "used youth at once to denounce change and adapt to it."[6] This chapter will explore how adult concerns about the shifting social order influenced scientific and popular understanding of what constituted "normal" adolescent development from the early twentieth century onward and the ways in which these developmental norms were shaped by gender. Historically, women have been subjected to more medical scrutiny than men due to beliefs that the female body was inherently pathological. As Carroll Smith-Rosenberg observes in her classic essay "Puberty to Menopause," medical theories about women's bodies both reflected and reinforced notions of women's proper roles. Medical experts claimed women were "prisoners" of their reproductive systems, with the onset of puberty being the greatest "crisis" in a woman's life. If a girl did not observe the laws of hygiene at puberty, she would suffer menstrual disorders, infertility, and medical problems.[7]

During the first half of the twentieth century, experts in child development invented new techniques for measuring growth and assessing pubertal development. The growing professional authority of medicine ensured that deviation from accepted physical and psychological norms would be regarded as an illness that required treatment by trained medical experts. As the power and prestige of the medical profession grew during the first half of the twentieth century, various forms of deviance, such as alcoholism and homosexuality, were transformed from being "bad behaviors" into "sicknesses" that necessitated medical intervention.[8] This chapter will examine how this process of medicalization shaped pediatric medicine. Children and adolescents who did not fit standardized norms of physical and mental development became targets of new medical treatments, especially if their bodies did not conform to prevailing norms about masculinity and femininity.

The emergence of child study as a scientific field at the turn of the twentieth century intersected with broader social concerns about the impact of modern urban industrial life on young people's health. The cultural historian T. J. Jackson Lears has used the term "antimodernism" to describe this sentiment.[9] In his monumental 1904 book, *Adolescence: Its Psychology and Its Relation to Physiology, Anthropology, Sociology, Sex, Crime, Religion, and Education*, the child study pioneer G. Stanley Hall incorporated this antimodernist sentiment into a theory of adolescent development. He drew together existing studies on adolescent development and placed them within the framework of evolutionary biology. The central concept of Hall's theory of human development was the notion that ontogeny recapitulated phylogeny: that is, each stage of human development reiterated specific periods in the evolution of the human race. According to Hall, adolescence corresponded to an ancient period of "storm and stress," during which "the floodgates of heredity seemed opened and we hear from our remoter forebears." Hall's image of adolescence as "the paradise of the race from which adult life is a fall" appealed to those who, like Hall, feared modern industrial society was "at root morbific and sure to end in reaction and decay." Hall argued that in order to reach healthy maturity, adolescents had to be protected from the "overcivilization" of the adult world and instead emulate the deeds and sentiments of their more "primitive" ancestors.[10]

Hall's warnings about the dangers of "overcivilization" for adolescents led to a variety of social reforms aimed at improving the health and welfare of the nation's children and youth. To many early twentieth-century reformers, Hall's theory of recapitulation provided the scientific basis for child labor laws, compulsory schooling, playgrounds, youth clubs, and other institutions for young people. Reformers portrayed children and adolescents as innocent, immature beings who needed protection from the dangers of the adult world. The legitimacy of pediatrics as a distinct medical specialty was bolstered by these reform efforts. Pediatricians not only were critical to advancing these child-saving initiatives but also used them to justify their claims to specialized knowledge in the health care of children.[11]

Medical experts warned parents about the dangers of children who assumed adult roles and responsibilities at too young an age. Parents were advised against sending their sons to college or into the workforce before they had sufficient judgment to resist adult temptations.[12] Physicians claimed that "precocious" intellectual development could lead to other unacceptable behaviors, most notably masturbation. Although physicians argued that masturbation was harmful at all ages, they believed it was especially dangerous during puberty since it hindered physical and mental development.[13]

Warnings about the dangers of precocious development were even stronger for girls because of a growing gap between sexual maturation and marriage. The average age of first menstruation in the late nineteenth century was sixteen, but medical experts recommended that women should not marry until their mid-twenties, when they had developed sufficient strength for childbearing. Historian Joan Jacobs Brumberg describes how parents and physicians attempted to alleviate the sexual dangers posed by this "new timetable" and even delay menarche "by restricting a girl's intake of foods that were considered sexually 'stimulating,' such as cloves, pickles, and meat." Brumberg shows how reformers at this time created a "protective umbrella" over female adolescence by establishing single-sex groups such as the Girls Scouts, Campfire Girls, and the Young Women's Christian (or Hebrew) Association "devoted to the common mission of keeping girlhood wholesome and chaste." During the 1880s, the Woman's Christian Temperance Union began a nationwide campaign to raise the age of consent from a low of ten in some states to sixteen. These led to the creation of statutory rape laws aimed at "protecting innocent girls from the vices of adult men."[14]

Concerns about the dangers of precocity served to justify mandatory schooling through high school for both boys and girls. As a result, school attendance by adolescents aged fourteen through sixteen increased from 6.7 percent in 1890 to over 50 percent by the 1930s. At the same time, schools organized students into grades determined by age group rather than academic achievement. Many school districts also created junior high schools that separated pubescent girls and boys from older and younger students and further narrowed their institutional peer groupings.[15]

Hall cautioned against educating the sexes together because of a notable gap between the ages at which boys and girls reached puberty. Earlier studies of Boston-area schoolchildren conducted by Henry P. Bowditch, professor of physiology at Harvard Medical School, found significant sex differences in the maturation of boys and girls. Until the age of eleven or twelve, boys were both taller and heavier than girls of the same age. After age twelve, girls began their growth spurt and for the next two or three years were taller and heavier than boys in their age group. After boys finished their growth spurt, they achieved a superior height and weight than girls. Bowditch wondered whether it was appropriate to educate boys and girls together given the marked gap between male and female growth spurts.[16] Hall did his doctoral work with Bowditch and elaborated on these concerns. Because boys were further "from the nubile maturity" than female classmates of their own age, said Hall, intimate daily contact between boys and girls would cause boys to assert their manhood in a "premature and excessive" manner. This could lead to marriage that violated "the important physiological law of disparity that requires the husband to be some years the wife's senior." For girls, constant interaction with "underdeveloped" boys of her own age might lead to "mute disenchantment" with men and a disinclination toward marriage.[17]

Single-sex education proved to be impractical for most public schools. Instead, public schools tracked girls into separate curricula such as home economics. This academic segregation was bolstered by medical claims that excessive intellectual demands could impede girls' physical development. Drawing on conservation of energy principles, Hall argued that the brain withdrew physical energy from the rest of the body during intellectual activities. Although this principle applied to both sexes, Hall claimed the development of the female reproductive system was more likely to be derailed by excessive mental strain and that women's health was "even more important for the welfare of the race than that of man." Institutions charged with educating girls during adolescence, "when the period most favorable to motherhood begins," should follow "the cult of the goddess Hygeia" by requiring students to follow the latest recommendations in nutrition, sleep, exercise, and other advances in "health culture."[18]

Hall's chief accomplishment was to establish the scientific field of child study, yet his work also ensured that the medical treatment of children and adolescents would evolve along distinctly gendered lines. During the first half of the twentieth century, child study researchers accumulated data on thousands of children and adolescents and used these to create standardized growth charts that indicated the average height and weight for a particular age. This information was incorporated into the pediatric curriculum and used to justify the expansion of pediatrics into well-child care. Pediatricians argued that they should not only treat children when they were sick but also provide regular checkups to ensure they were developing normally. Children who were below average for height and weight might have underlying diseases that needed medical treatment.[19] According to historians Janet Golden and Russell M. Viner, "by the mid-twentieth century, weighing and measuring had become a ritual" in both public clinics and private practice. This "standardization" grew out of "the belief that poorly grown and undernourished children could be identified before they became sick" and without intervention "would later be unfit for work or military service in the case of boys, and for motherhood, in the case of girls." These new standards of normality represented "the extension of medical supervision into new areas of childhood, the redefinition of normality in statistical and clinical terms, and a shifting locus of judgment from family and peers to clinicians."[20]

This information about "normal" growth and development was disseminated to the public through advice manuals, Better Babies and Better Families contests, exhibits at state fairs, public school hygiene courses, and popular articles and pamphlets. Public schoolchildren learned about human growth through classroom activities designed to make science interesting and relevant to everyday life.[21] Yet it was unclear what these growth standards really meant.

Could a child be "normal" if he or she was not "average"? Mothers panicked when their children did not develop "on schedule."[22] Children and adolescents also worried about how they "measured up" to standardized growth charts.[23]

Confusion about what was "normal" development reflected the limitations of the growth studies conducted in the 1920s and the 1930s, which used a cross-sectional method based on the belief that growth followed a uniform, biologically determined progression. Thus, researchers believed that taking an average of various individuals of the same age was sufficient for charting normal development.[24] Beginning in the 1930s, child development researchers realized that longitudinal studies of child and adolescent growth were needed in order to more accurately evaluate whether an individual's growth was "normal." One of the leaders in this endeavor was Laurence K. Frank, associate director of the Laura Spelman Rockefeller Memorial and, later, the General Education Board of the Rockefeller Foundation, which were leading funders of child development research in the mid-twentieth century. Frank criticized the "tyranny of the norm" imposed by standardized height and weight charts and believed they had especially dire consequences for adolescents who were more obsessed with their normality than other age groups.[25]

Developmental studies conducted in the 1930s and 1940s revealed there was considerable variation in the age of onset of puberty and rate of growth during adolescence. Since these studies started during the Great Depression, researchers were especially interested in determining the impact of economic deprivation on child growth. These studies also made a distinction between "chronological age" and "physiological age." The term "physiological age" was first used in 1908 by school physician C. Ward Crampton, who sought a way to determine fitness for school athletics that was more accurate than chronological age.[26] Researchers used newly developed techniques in radiology to find a specific marker for physiological age. The first efforts to do so were done under the supervision of T. Wingate Todd at the Brush Foundation at Case Western Reserve University in Cleveland. Todd argued that skeletal maturation was a more objective measure of physical maturation than height or weight. According to Todd, each child followed a "time clock" of skeletal development. Although individual children could arrive at developmental milestones at different ages, they all went through the same sequence. In 1937, Todd published his *Atlas of Skeletal Maturation*, which contained a system for grading physiological age according to the development of bones in the hand, wrist, and knees.[27] Like Hall, Todd commented on the "adolescent lag," or difference in growth of boys and girls of the same chronological age. Although Todd believed it was normal for girls to experience their growth spurt first, the "adolescent lag" could have serious psychological consequences for boys. Todd suggested grouping students based on physiological age rather than chronological age to prevent feelings of inferiority in boys who felt overwhelmed by girls who were physically larger than them.[28]

Todd's scale was further refined by his successors at Case Western, William Greulich and Idell Pyle, whose radiographic atlas became the standard diagnostic tool for assessing physiological age.[29] Greulich also began the first investigations into the relationship between the development of secondary sexual characteristics and hormone secretions during adolescence and was the first to outline stages of sexual maturity as shown by development of the genitalia.[30] These stages of sexual development were further developed by Herbert and Lois Stolz at the University of California, Berkeley and by Earle Reynolds at the Fels Research Institute at Antioch College.[31]

Although developmental researchers attempted to expand the understanding of what constituted normal development, they also recognized that adolescents who differed significantly from their peers could have emotional problems. "One of the greatest obstacles to social acceptance is being different," Herbert and Lois Stolz wrote. Adolescents were especially disturbed by bodily features that deviated from culturally accepted physical characteristics for men and women. For boys, short stature was the most frequent problem that caused emotional distress. Boys also worried about "feminine" physical features such as excessive accumulation of fat around the hips and thighs. For girls, "excessive" height was the most common complaint, followed by delayed appearance of breasts and excessive, "masculine" muscle development. The Stolzes argued that most cases of apparent physical abnormality were a "passing phase" on the road to normal development and that "sympathetic guidance" from pediatricians, parents, and teachers would lead to "social acceptance and self-acceptance."[32]

The emerging field of pediatric endocrinology offered new approaches to addressing problems of adolescent growth. The first pediatric endocrinology clinic in the country was established at Johns Hopkins University in 1935, with Lawson Wilkins as director.[33] As the general public became aware of hormonal treatments through coverage in the popular press, pediatric endocrinologists found themselves consulted by parents of otherwise healthy children whose growth lagged behind their peers. In his textbook on pediatric endocrinology published in 1950, Lawson Wilkins warned his colleagues to resist demands from parents who were "frequently alarmed and excessively worried because they have been told by well-meaning friends, teachers, or doctors that the child has a 'glandular disorder.'" Caving to such demands not only resulted in "needless therapy" but could also "give rise to psychologic difficulties in the future" by fixing the idea of abnormality in the child's mind. Wilkins was especially adamant about the overdiagnosis of Frölich's syndrome, a pituitary disorder that caused obesity, sluggishness, and delayed sexual development in boys. Wilkins argued that the diagnosis should never be made unless there was a proven lesion and that most fat boys with delayed sexual development would eventually mature normally. Yet Wilkins acknowledged that there were some cases "in which delayed adolescence in boys leads to psychologic inferiority so serious as to justify endocrine therapy." Wilkins also presented the pros and cons of using hormone treatment to treat "unusually tall" girls. Although he recognized that "excessive tallness" was a handicap for girls, he warned that hormonal treatment "might interfere with establishment of normal menstrual cycles" and jeopardize their ability to have children later in life.[34]

The new information on adolescent growth and development that emerged from these studies made the pediatrician's job more challenging. No longer could pediatricians simply compare children to a standard height and weight chart. Instead, growth assessment involved plotting the individual child's growth patterns from birth and determining whether the tempo of growth was appropriate for that child based on earlier data. If a child appeared to be accelerating or lagging in growth rate as compared to previous trends, he or she might need referral to a specialist in pediatric endocrinology.

The child development studies conducted in the United States served as inspiration for James Mourilyan Tanner and Reginald H. Whitehouse's groundbreaking longitudinal study of English schoolchildren conducted at the Harpenden National Children's Home between 1949 and 1971.[35] The study examined 450 boys and 260 girls from the age of three or four. Most of the children were white, although there were a few subjects who were of African descent. Tanner and Whitehouse were especially interested in studying growth during puberty. During the study, they measured and photographed 228 boys and 192 girls every three months as they went through puberty. They used manual palpation to assess the emergence of breast tissue and a tool known as an orchidometer to measure testicular development. These measurements were then compiled and analyzed and used to create the Tanner scale of pubertal changes that is now used by clinicians to measure and describe the development of pubic hair, breasts (for girls), and testes and penis (for boys). This scale was first published in 1962 and has since become the standard against which pediatricians assess sexual maturation of children and adolescents.[36]

Another key finding of Tanner's research was that the average age of puberty in Europe and the United States had declined significantly over the previous century. In a 1966 article entitled "The Earlier Maturation of Children," published in the British publication *Nursing Mirror and Midwife Journal*, Tanner described what he called a "secular trend," that is, a notable decline in the average age of puberty over time. He mentioned studies of female hospital patients in Oslo, Norway, in the 1850s who experienced first menstruation at the "to us, astonishing late age of 17." Other data from Norway regarding the growth rates of young men indicated that on average, they reached their maximum growth velocity at seventeen or eighteen. According to Tanner, "as the average peak velocity of boys' height growth is reached about one year after the average menarche of girls, this is in complete agreement with menarche data." Further studies in Norway showed that the age of menarche had fallen to fifteen by 1910. Data from other parts of Europe indicated a similar "secular trend" in the age of menarche. Tanner charted a continued rate of fall of about one year per generation, resulting in an average age of 13 in Great Britain and 12.6 or 12.7 among the "well-off classes" in the United States. Tanner claimed that "there is no evidence the trend is stopping, or that girls are now reaching maturity at the earliest possible time." In fact, he said, "we may expect the fall to continue for at least another 20 to 30 years."[37]

News of Tanner's results soon entered the American popular science press. In a *Scientific American* article entitled "Earlier Maturation in Man" (1968). Tanner described the trend toward earlier maturation, which was "best shown by statistics on the age of menarche," which had "fallen considerably over the previous century." Tanner admitted that earlier records of age at menarche suffered from "disadvantages of both sampling and technique." Most of those collected prior to 1920 involved hospital patients and relied on recollections of women interviewed ten to thirty years after they first menstruated. "In spite of such defects," Tanner argued, the data on menarcheal age were "remarkably consistent" across time and place, and the main conclusion was "perfectly clear: girls have experienced menarche progressively earlier during the past 100 years." Tanner attributed this decline largely to environmental factors, such as improved nutrition and decline in the incidence of childhood diseases. He also tried to dismiss common misconceptions about the possible causes of the declining age of menarche. He discredited the classic view that menarche occurred earlier in warmer climates, observing that while the mean world temperature had been increasing since the 1850s, it seemed "unlikely on present evidence" that this warming tendency had "contributed significantly to the trend toward earlier menarche." He also dispelled the suggestion that "an increasing emphasis on sex" and psychosocial stimulation among boys and girls was to blame. Tanner noted that comparisons of European schoolgirls educated in single-sex and coeducational schools showed no difference in age of onset of menstruation.

Whether these studies were a "fair test of school-days sex activity" remained to be seen, he said, but should "psychosocial sexual stimulation actually be the cause" of earlier maturation, "it would have to start in nursery school."[38]

Data about the earlier age of puberty in boys were more difficult to pin down, since boys did not have a specific biological marker like menarche to signal this change. Tanner said that appearance of pubic hair was not as reliable an indicator as first menstruation, and there were insufficient historical data to track change over time. The most dependable source was a study at Oxford that compared the age at which modern choir boys' voices "broke"—that is, fell to a lower register—with those of Johann Sebastian Bach's Leipzig choir in the eighteenth century. This study found that in Bach's day, the average age at which boys stopped singing soprano was 18, while boys in the 1950s had an average age of voice change of 13.3.[39]

News about the secular trend soon became accepted popular wisdom, feeding into preexisting fears about the impact of modern life on children and the imminent "disappearance" of childhood.[40] Some popular news accounts claimed that this secular trend was the main cause of the sexual revolution among young people and a growing "epidemic" of teenage pregnancy. "What looks like a new morality is a new biology," Dr. Andre E. Hellegers of Georgetown University Medical School told the *Boston Globe* in 1973. This "new biology" was especially dangerous for girls, he observed. "Parents lie awake at night in suburban homes at midnight when their 13-year-old daughter is out babysitting," he said. "They worry about the girl being sexually assaulted."[41] Some argued that early puberty increased the likelihood that a child would become homosexual. According to social psychologist Michael D. Storms of the University of Kansas, children who matured prematurely when they were in single-sex social groups learned "from an environment rich in homosexual cues." Children who matured later, when boys and girls were "more integrated socially," tended "to eroticize heterosexual cues and to develop an ultimate preference for heterosexual relationships."[42]

Thus, the current sense of "crisis" about an earlier timetable for sexual maturation is not new but has a long history dating back to the early twentieth century. Like earlier commentators, medical scientists and popular science writers today attribute declining age of puberty to a host of modern social ills, including pesticides, hormones in meat and milk, obesity, and sexualized messages in the media.[43] More recent studies of early puberty, though, employ a different metric than earlier reports. Instead of tracing the age of menstruation or voice change, these researchers use the Tanner stages that had been incorporated into pediatric training on adolescent development. According to Tanner's guidelines, the average age for children reaching Tanner stage 2 was eleven, and the lowest "normal" age for Tanner was eight years of age for girls and nine years of age for boys. Children who reached this stage earlier than these standard ages were referred to pediatric endocrinologists for assessment to see if they had hormonal imbalances or tumors that might be affecting their development.[44]

Herman-Giddens's work suggesting that girls and boys might be exhibiting the early stages of puberty as young as six or seven created a stir in a popular press that had already spent decades reporting on the secular trend. Notably, the majority (three-quarters) of popular articles published in the wake of Herman-Giddens's results highlighted the data on girls.[45] This very fact indicates a cultural preoccupation with the sexual dangers associated with the declining age of puberty in girls. *New York Times* health columnist Jane Brody started an article on Herman-Giddens's study entitled "Yesterday's Precocious Puberty Is Norm Today" with a comment on teenage mothers. "While children having children is not a new phenomenon," she observed, "the ever-dropping age of puberty is." Brody argued that early maturing girls needed "explicit sex education," since adults who delayed educating girls would "end up with pregnant 13-year olds."[46] Other reports indicated that early maturing girls were more vulnerable to depression, anxiety, and low self-esteem.[47] Cancer researchers proposed a link between early puberty and breast cancer.[48] Discussions of the causes of the "new puberty" in girls also reflect cultural anxieties about gender roles and family relationships. For example, some researchers reported that the absence of a biological father in the home correlated with early puberty in girls.[49]

Articles on boys suggested that those who start puberty early may exhibit aggressive or antisocial behaviors. In general, though, boys themselves viewed early puberty in positive terms, and parents were proud of sons who were larger and more muscular than other boys.[50] Some articles tended to focus on the negative impact of girls' earlier age of puberty on boys' self-esteem. For example, an article from the *Chicago Tribune* entitled "Keeping Up with the Girls" observed, "As if boys in elementary and middle school didn't already have enough ways to compare themselves unfavorably with girls—scholastic achievement, verbal skills and social prowess, not to mention handwriting and knowledge about horses—this trend toward precocious sexual development just may be the final nail in the coffin of male domination."[51]

Herman-Giddens's work also touched off a debate among pediatric endocrinologists about the best way to treat precocious puberty. Some pediatric endocrinologists argued that Herman-Giddens's work was flawed because it was not drawn from a random sample of the general population and was therefore apt to have ascertainment bias. They argued that "liberalizing the definition of nor-mal" risked overlooking serious underlying medical conditions that could be causing early puberty. In addition, they suggested that precocious puberty in and of itself was a disease that needed to be cured with synthetic gonadotro-pin-releasing hormone agonists (GnRHA), marketed under the tradename Lupron. Left untreated, these experts argued, precocious puberty could lead to serious psychosocial consequences, such as low self-esteem, depression, con-duct disorders, and early drug use and sexual activity.[52] Endocrinologists observed that children with precocious puberty finished their growth spurt ear-lier and thus had a lower adult height than they would have had puberty arrived "on schedule." They claimed the psychological effects of short stature were especially dire for boys given the correlation between height and profes-sional success later in life. Some doctors also began using Lupron "off-label" to forestall puberty so that a child's final adult height would be higher. Delaying puberty solely for the purpose of increasing final height was controversial among some pediatric endocrinologists, though. One noted that "adolescence is hard enough when everything is going right"; boys whose puberty was delayed in order to increase their final height would have undeveloped genitalia well into middle school and could face ridicule and bulling from their larger peers.[53]

Other pediatric endocrinologists suggested that Herman-Giddens's study should be used to set new age limits for when puberty was truly "precocious." In 1999, Dr. Paul Kaplowitz, a pediatric endocrinologist at the Medical College of Virginia, and Dr. Sharon Oberfield, a pediatric endocrinologist at Columbia University College of Physicians and Surgeons, published a paper suggesting that most children who developed secondary sexual characteristics before age eight or nine should be considered normal and should not be treated with Lupron to delay puberty.[54] Kaplowitz incorporated these recommendations in a clinical report for the section on endocrinology of the American Academy of Pediatrics aimed at providing advice to primary care practitioners. The report observes that while early onset of puberty "may be a sign of a serious underly-ing disorder requiring therapy, the majority of cases, especially in girls, are benign, normal variants that do not require extensive testing or treatment." The article acknowledged that in some cases, there were "justifiable reasons" for drug treatment. One of these was "the preservation of height potential." Other reasons included "prevention of early menarche and the psychological ramifi-cations that accompany it," especially for girls with developmental disabilities, and "suppression of sexual maturation in a girl who is emotionally immature." Yet Lupron was expensive—$15,000 or more per year—"so the decision to treat should not be taken lightly."[55]

Treatment with Lupron not only is costly but can also cause serious medical problems. The common short-term effects include mood changes, acne, excessive facial hair, and breakthrough vaginal bleeding, which for some children can be more distressing than early puberty itself. Long-term health problems include premature bone thinning, osteoporosis, depression, anxiety, and polycystic ovarian syndrome in girls and young women.[56] Nevertheless, many parents are opting for treatment in order to diminish the psychosocial consequences of early sexual development and ensure that a child achieves his or her maximum adult height. Historically, shortness was considered bad for boys, while being "too tall" was considered a "handicap" for girls. Now our society's preference for taller bodies includes girls as well. This contributes to our society's "heightism," or discrimination based on height, and because the cost of treatment is so high, ensures that lower-income children will be more likely to suffer from this form of social prejudice.

Managing the "problem" of early puberty also includes addressing the threats of other health issues later in life. As in the past, the long-term health consequences of early puberty are believed to be especially bad for girls. Medical experts claim that early breast development makes girls more susceptible to breast cancer, while girls who develop pubic hair early may be more at risk for metabolic disorders such as obesity, diabetes, and heart disease.[57] This continues a longer tradition of heightened medical scrutiny of female bodies from puberty to menopause and beyond.

More recently, pediatricians have encountered the ethical and medical issues surrounding the treatment of transgendered children and adolescents. Gonadotropin-releasing hormone (GnRH) and other puberty blockers created to treat precocious puberty are now being increasingly used "off-label" to delay puberty in children who identify as transgender or who are gender nonconforming. In their article "New Puberty, New Trans: Children, Pharmaceuticals and Politics," Celia Roberts and Cron Cronshaw observe that these therapies have been "hailed by clinicians, parents, therapists and trans young people and adults as a lifesaving option" because they allow children to avoid "the psychological suffering involved in living through an unwanted sexual development." Roberts and Cronshaw see these remedies as part of a longer process of medicalization of childhood, using the term "pharmaceuticalization" to describe the growing use of "pharmaceuticals to address experiences and bodies previously lived outside of medical regimes." Although they agree that treating trans children with puberty blockers "may provide much-needed breathing space for young people," these treatments are based on "an underlying assumption of binary gender" and enforce "conventional figurations of sex/gender." By treating trans children to conform to a normative distinction between male and female, they argue, clinicians marginalize children and adults who do not conform to this gender binary (including genderqueer, nongendered, intersex, and transgendered persons who decline surgery or hormonal treatment). They conclude that medical interventions for trans children are driven less by the child's own interests and more by "adults' desires for clarity about a child's sex/gender and future."[58] Therefore, this new approach to trans children, like the "new puberty" before it, is the product of adult anxieties about child development and our society's discomfort with bodies that do not fit within accepted biological norms.

Notes

1. Marcia Herman-Giddens et al., "Secondary Sexual Characteristics and Menses in Young Girls Seen in Office Practice: A Study from the Pediatric Research in Office Settings Network," *Pediatrics* 99, no. 4 (1997): 505–12.
2. Marcia Herman-Giddens et al., "Secondary Sexual Characteristics in Boys: Estimates from the National Health and Nutrition Examination Survey III, 1988–1994," *Archives of Pediatric and Adolescent Medicine* 155 (2001): 1022–28.
3. Louise Greenspan and Julianna Deardorf, *The New Puberty: How to Navigate Early Development in Today's Girls* (New York: Rodale, 2014).
4. Lisa Belkin, "The Making of an 8-Year-Old Woman," *New York Times Magazine,* December 24, 2000, 38–43.
5. Celia Roberts, *Puberty in Crisis: The Sociology of Early Sexual Development* (Cambridge: Cambridge University Press, 2015), 1.
6. Paula Fass, *The Damned and the Beautiful: American Youth in the 1920s* (New York: Oxford University Press, 1977), 234.
7. Carroll Smith-Rosenberg, "Puberty to Menopause: The Cycle of Femininity in Nineteenth-Century America," *Feminist Studies* 1 (1973): 58–72.
8. Peter Conrad and Joseph W. Schneider, *Deviance and Medicalization: From Badness to Sickness* (St. Louis, MO: Mosby, 1980).
9. Jackson Lears, *No Place of Grace: Antimodernism and the Transformation of American Culture, 1890–1920* (New York: Pantheon Books, 1981).
10. G. Stanley Hall, *Adolescence: Its Psychology and Its Relation to Physiology, Anthropology, Sociology, Sex, Crime, Religion, and Education,* vol. II (New York: D. Appleton, 1904), 747. For more on Hall's life and work, see Dorothy Ross, *G. Stanley Hall: The Psychologist as Prophet* (Chicago: University of Chicago Press, 1972).
11. Sydney Halpern, *American Pediatrics: The Social Dynamics of Professionalism, 1880–1980* (Berkeley: University of California Press, 1988).
12. Joseph Kett, *Rites of Passage: Adolescence in America, 1790 to the Present* (New York: Basic Books, 1977), 215–44.
13. Arthur N. Gilbert, "Doctor, Patient, and Onanist Diseases in the Nineteenth Century," *Journal of the History of Medicine and Allied Sciences* 30, no. 3 (1975): 217–34.
14. Joan Jacobs Brumberg, *The Body Project: An Intimate History of American Girls* (New York: Random House, 1997), 10–11, 16–17.
15. Howard P. Chudacoff, *How Old Are You? Age Consciousness in American Culture* (Princeton, NJ: Princeton University Press, 1989), 98–99.

16. James M. Tanner, *A History of the Study of Human Growth* (Cambridge: Cambridge University Press, 1981), 189–94.

17. Hall, *Adolescence*, vol. II, 626–27.

18. Hall, *Adolescence*, vol. II, 631, 637.

19. Sydney Halpern, *American Pediatrics: The Social Dynamics of Professionalism, 1880–1980* (Berkeley: University of California Press, 1988), 80–109.

20. Russell Viner and Janet Golden, "Children's Experiences of Illness," in *Medicine in the Twentieth Century*, ed. Roger Cooter and John Pickstone (Amsterdam: Harwood Academic, 2000), 582–83.

21. Elizabeth Toon, "Measuring Up: Educators, Schoolchildren, and Representations of Physical Growth in the Interwar U.S.," paper presented at the annual meeting of the History of Science Society, Vancouver, British Columbia, November 3, 2000.

22. Julia Grant, *Raising Baby by the Book: The Education of American Mothers* (New Haven, CT: Yale University Press, 1998), 215–18.

23. Brumberg, *The Body Project*; Elizabeth Toon and Janet Golden, "Rethinking Charles Atlas," *Rethinking History* 4, no. 1 (2000): 80–84.

24. Tanner, *Human Growth*, 244.

25. Lawrence K. Frank, "Certain Problems of Puberty and Adolescence," *Journal of Pediatrics* 19 (1941): 296.

26. Tanner, *Human Growth*, 244.

27. T. Wingate Todd, *Atlas of Skeletal Maturation* (London: Kimpton, 1937).

28. T. Wingate Todd, "The Adolescent Lag," in *Physical and Mental Adolescent Growth: The Proceedings of the Conference on Adolescence, Cleveland, Ohio, October 17 and 18, 1930* (Cleveland, OH: Brush Foundation, 1931), 1–4.

29. William W. Greulich and S. Idell Pyle, *Radiographic Atlas of Skeletal Development of the Hand and Wrist* (Palo Alto, CA: Stanford University Press, 1950).

30. William W. Greulich, *Somatic and Endocrine Studies of Pubertal and Adolescent Boys*, Monographs of the Society for Research in Child Development, 7, no. 3 (serial no. 33), 1942.

31. Herbert Rowell Stolz and Lois Meek Stolz, *Somatic Development of Adolescent Boys* (New York: Macmillan, 1951); Earle L. Reynods and J. V. Vines, "Individual Differences in Physical Changes Associated with Adolescence in Girls," *American Journal of Diseases of Children* 75 (1948): 329–50; Earle L. Reynolds and J. V. Vines, "Physical Changes Associated with Adolescence in Boys," *American Journal of Diseases of Children* 82 (1951): 529–47.

32. Herbert R. Stolz and Lois M. Stolz, "Adolescent Problems Related to Somatic Variations," in *Forty-Third Yearbook of the National Society for the Study of Education, Pt. 1, Adolescence*, ed. Henry Nelson Bollinger (Chicago: University of Chicago Press, 1944), 80–99.

33. Halpern, *American Pediatrics*, 115.

34. Lawson Wilkins, *The Diagnosis and Treatment of Endocrine Disorders in Childhood and Adolescence* (Springfield, IL: Charles C Thomas, 1950), 141–44.

35. Nöel Cameron, "The Human Biology of Jim Tanner," *Annals of Human Biology* 5, no. 39 (2012): 329–34.

36. James M. Tanner, *Growth at Adolescence* (Springfield, IL: Thomas, 1962). For more on the history of the Tanner scale, see Roberts, *Puberty in Crisis*, 51–90.

37. James M. Tanner, "The Earlier Maturation of Children," *Nursing Mirror and Midwife Journal* 121, no. 169 (1966): 21–22.

38. James M. Tanner, "Earlier Maturation in Man," *Scientific American* 218, no. 1 (1968): 21–27.

39. Walter Sullivan, "Boys and Girls Are Now Maturing Earlier, Scientists Find," *New York Times*, January 24, 1971, 1.

40. Neil Postman, *The Disappearance of Childhood* (New York: Delacorte Press, 1982); Marie Winn, *Children without Childhood* (New York: Penguin, 1982).

41. Stuart Auerbach, "Early Sexual Maturity Poses Problem," *Boston Globe*, September 6, 1973, 33.

42. W. Herbert, "Homosexuality Roots: Precocious Puberty?" *Science News* 122 (September 4, 1982): 151.

43. Belkin, "The Making of an 8-Year-Old Woman."

44. Roberts, *Puberty in Crisis*, 96.

45. Sharon R. Mazzerella, "Coming of Age Too Soon: Journalistic Practice in U.S. Newspaper Coverage of 'Early Puberty' in Girls," *Communication Quarterly* 58, no. 1 (2010): 36–58.

46. Jane E. Brody, "Yesterday's Precocious Puberty Is Norm Today," *New York Times*, November 30, 1999: F, 8:1.

47. Perri Klass, "Earlier Puberty in Girls Raises the Risk of Depression," *New York Times*, June 6, 2016.

48. The link between early puberty and breast cancer is being investigated by the Bay-Area research study Cohort of Young Girls' Nutrition, Environment, and Transitions (CYGNET), http://cygnetstudy.com/about-cygnet/history (accessed January 8, 2019).

49. Bruce J. Ellis et al., "Quality of Early Family Relationships and Individual Differences in the Timing of Pubertal Maturation in Girls: A Longitudinal Test of an Evolutionary Model," *Journal of Personality and Social Psychology* 77, no. 2 (1999): 387–401.

50. Tara Parker-Pope, "Rise in Early Puberty Causes Parents to Ask, 'When Is It Too Soon?'" *Wall Street Journal*, July 21, 2000, B1.

51. Meghan Daum, "Keeping Up with the Girls," *Chicago Tribune*, August 13, 2010, 17.

52. Robert L. Rosenfield et al., "Letter to the Editor: Current Age of Onset of Puberty," *Pediatrics* 106 (2000): 622.

53. Susan Cohen and Christine Cosgrove, *Normal at Any Cost: Tall Girls, Short Boys, and the Medical Industry's Quest to Manipulate Height* (New York: Jeremy P. Tarcher/Penguin, 2009), 195–96.

54. Paul B. Kaplowitz and Sharon E. Oberfield, "Reexamination of the Age Limit for Defining When Puberty Is Precocious in Girls in the United States: Implications for Evaluation and Treatment. Drug and Therapeutics and Executive Committees of the Lawson Wilkins Pediatric Endocrine Society," *Pediatrics* 104 (1999): 936–41.

55. Paul Kaplowitz and Clifford Bloch, "Evaluation and Referral of Children with Signs of Early Puberty," *Pediatrics* 137, no. 1 (January 2016): 1–6.

56. Christina Jewett, "Women Fear Drug They Used to Halt Puberty Led to Health Problems," Kaiser Health News, February 2, 2017, https://khn.org/news/women-fear-drug-they-used-to-halt-puberty-led-to-health-problems (accessed January 25, 2019).

57. Greenspan and Deardorf, *The New Puberty*, 81.

58. Celia Roberts and Cron Cronshaw, "New Puberty; New Trans: Children, Pharmaceuticals and Politics," in *Gendering Drugs: Feminist Studies of Pharmaceuticals*, ed. Erick Johnson (Cham, Switzerland: Palgrave Macmillan, 2017), 60, 70, 73, 81.

Chapter 11

Gender and HPV Vaccination

Responsible Boyhood or Responsible Girls and Women?

Laura Mamo and Ashley E. Pérez

Something remarkable has happened to the human papillomavirus (HPV) vaccine since its introduction in 2006: what began as a charged set of conversations around sex, gender, and responsibility gradually settled and then shifted as new guidelines, groups, and professionals became involved in vaccination efforts.[1] Today, HPV vaccination is a largely settled public health strategy to protect girls from cervical cancer in adulthood, and guidelines explicitly include boys and all young people in the effort. However, public concerns linger regarding what the virus is, what other health risks it poses, and for whom, revealing cultural uneasiness, if not uncertainty, about the vaccine. This chapter analyzes the ways gendering, degendering and regendering processes have variously punctuated the trajectory of HPV vaccination in the United States. We argue that a regendering of HPV and HPV cancer prevention has taken place through an alignment with femininity and cisgender women's bodies. We examine HPV vaccination policy, pharma advertising, and organizational and popular media to draw attention to temporal shifts that have led to the recent hard public and pediatric sell of an all-gender approach.

In doing so, we show that just as gender inclusion moves toward a settled policy and practice approach for HPV vaccination, a renewed gendered responsibility for cancer prevention is gradually, and simultaneously, emerging in calls for "vaccination plus screening" approaches to HPV-related cancer prevention. These calls, we argue, serve to regender HPV in their alignment with women's health infrastructures and gendered expectations. While adolescent boys and some men are shaped as innocent actors able to—with support from a collective of women—contribute to population health, and gay men and other men who have sex with men (MSM) are advocating for disease prevention, cisgender girls and women continue to hold the burden for cancer prevention through primary vaccination plus secondary screening prevention tools that conjoin as the newly established "right tool" for cervical cancer prevention.

Echoing the case of the male contraceptive pill studied by Nelly Oudshoorn,[2] our analysis shows that an alignment of "femininity" with HPV and HPV prevention needed to first be secured as girls were targeted as the early adopters of HPV vaccines. Then, as policy shifted and boys were enrolled in vaccination, this alignment needed to be supplanted by gender neutrality and processes of degendering. Finally, as we show, a realignment of femininity with HPV cancer prevention has reemerged with vaccination plus screening approaches, entangling pediatrics with adult care for women. Concomitantly, biomedicine and health care have undergone significant shifts from targeting illness to targeting health. As Clarke, Mamo, Fosket, Fishman, and Shim (2010) argue, "Health becomes an individual goal, a social and moral responsibility, and a site for routine biomedical intervention."[3] As biomedical processes travel beyond traditional medical domains and move culturally across airwaves, through collectives, and into public conversations, these shape publics as morally responsible for their own health. Gendering processes, as we show, are always and already entangled with other social categories such as age, sex and sexuality, and race/ethnicity in scientific claims-making as HPV and HPV vaccines are incorporated into policy guidelines and marketing approaches and taken up in media.[4]

The HPV Vaccine as the Right Tool for Cervical Cancer Prevention

The HPV vaccine entered public awareness and pediatric practice more than a decade ago through twenty-first-century direct-to-consumer (DTC) pharmaceutical disease awareness and advertising efforts. The vaccine, originally comprising three doses and approved for girls ages eleven to twelve with catchup vaccination up to age twenty-six, targeted four viral strains of a little-known sexually transmitted infection (STI), HPV, and its causal association with an uncommon but well-known cancer that affects people with cervices.[5] Prior to the vaccine's U.S. Food and Drug Administration (FDA) approval in 2006, the "right tool" for the job of cervical cancer prevention was the routinized and well-known Pap smear screening test used to detect precancerous lesions in adults with cervices, administered through gynecological health care, most often years after sexual debut.[6] This screening tool is recognized as having reduced cervical cancer by 70 percent in the United States.[7] But the new knowledge that these precancerous lesions were linked to HPV infection, combined with the technoscientific ability to produce virus-like particles and the promise of profitability, led pharma to invest in the development of an HPV vaccine.[8] Convincing the public that vaccination was the new "right tool" for cancer prevention, however, posed several challenges. One was to find ways to introduce a new approach to cancer prevention in the context of an already effective strategy known to most adults. Another was how to promote a new product without simultaneously drawing attention to gender and matters of sexual behavior.

The HPV vaccine entered public consciousness and implicated pediatrics when it was introduced as a vaccine targeting preadolescent and adolescent girls for a sexually transmitted virus that might, if a high-risk strain persists in the body, cause cancer. Uncertainty about the disease's causation and its association with sex and gender fueled an early challenge for Merck & Co., the HPV vaccine's first manufacturer: how to promote the vaccine without drawing attention to HPV's sexually transmitted nature. This was a particular concern given the age of the targeted population, preadolescent girls, whose sexuality is generally constructed as akin with innocence and in need of protection. In order to garner legitimacy, Merck discursively gendered and desexualized the vaccine by constructing cervical cancer, a cancer affecting women, rather than HPV, a ubiquitous STI, as the object of intervention.[9] Only one prior vaccine had been touted as a "cancer vaccine"—the hepatitis B vaccine, which, despite its early years including controversy surrounding its association with sex and MSM sexuality, became settled and universalized relatively early in its sociohistorical trajectory and is now part of newborn vaccination regimes.[10]

In 2005 and 2006, Merck's large-scale DTC awareness campaigns hit the airwaves and print advertising aiming to convince publics and pediatricians that "three shots of prevention" was the right tool for making girls *One Less* person with cervical cancer.[11] The *One Less* campaigns sought to enroll certain girls—responsible, self-reliant, at-risk individuals—to become the early adopters of a new approach to cancer prevention. They appealed directly to girls and their mothers to enroll girls in vaccination to reduce a silent killer affecting women. Producing a "will to knowledge" among girls, advertising suggested they had a responsibility to "know the link" between HPV and cervical cancer. Girls learned that they were bound together in a girlhood constructed as at risk yet self-responsible for collective education and action to secure future health.[12] In doing so, the HPV vaccine concretized the already present feminization of HPV by more directly associating the virus with cervical cancer, with cisgender girls, and with an already available feminization (and institutionalization) of the Pap test. Merck shifted cervical cancer risk from adult women, who had been encouraged to regularly seek cervical Pap testing, to presexual girls, now encouraged to join the American public in asking their doctors—in this case, their pediatricians—about a pharmaceutical approach, the Gardasil vaccine, to protect against future risk. Merck aligned the vaccine into already established discourses and consumer markets: a market of women aware of cervical cancer risk and their responsibility for prevention and a gendered public of women and girls responsible for reproductive and sexual health care.[13] A moral responsibility not only for one's health but for the collective health of the public was rhetorically mobilized by pharma and moved down the life course from women's "annual Pap" to empowered can-do girls.

Despite the widely distributed advertisements, by 2008 and 2009, 40.5 percent of U.S. girls between ages thirteen and seventeen had received at least one dose of the vaccine; 53.3 percent of them went on to complete the full three-dose series. There were notable racial disparities; Black and Latina girls were significantly less likely to have received the full vaccine series during these years.[14] Partly due to racial differences in Pap screening, stage at diagnosis, and follow-up after abnormal results, Black and Latina women were already disproportionately affected by HPV-associated cancers.[15] Public health responded with messages of individual responsibility, obfuscating the role of structural inequities and gaps in health care provision. Over time, adolescent vaccination became widely accepted for girls.[16] Further, vaccination gaps among Black and Latina girls began to close, even surpassing rates among white adolescents, which might ultimately help reduce racial disparities in cervical cancer.[17] However, feminization of the HPV vaccine inherently produced potential challenges to enrolling boys and men in vaccination in the coming years.

Degendering the HPV Vaccine: Producing Responsible Boyhood

In 2009, based on data from a clinical trial conducted in young men that found that HPV could lead to genital warts, the U.S. FDA approved use of the HPV vaccine in males ages nine to twenty-six, producing boys as at risk for genital warts from HPV.[18] The risk of genital warts seemed to offer a way for pharma and pediatrics to remedy boys' omission from HPV vaccination efforts and enjoin them in responsibility for health. However, unlike for girls and women, no formal *routine* vaccine recommendation was made. Rather, in 2009, the U.S. Centers for Disease Control and Prevention's Advisory Committee on Immunization Practices (ACIP) stated that the vaccine "*may* be given to males aged 9–26 years," leaving the decision to vaccinate up to professional judgment and publics with limited information on cancer and STI risks for boys.[19] This recommendation was based on knowledge that the vaccine could reduce risk of genital warts rather than cancer and that it would increase the population-level effectiveness of vaccination by reducing the number of people infected with HPV, thereby reducing onward transmission; universal vaccination would help to maximize the potential impact of vaccination for women, particularly prevention of cervical cancer. Although (binary) gender-neutral vaccination was introduced, evidence points to a pharma and pediatric narrative that wavered on whether boys and young men would be part of achieving herd immunity and constructed as responsible contributors to protecting people with cervices from a deadly cancer, as participants in a collective cancer prevention effort for all HPV-related cancers, or as direct recipients of individual protection against HPV-related disease.

In 2010, following the emergence of new evidence linking HPV to anal lesions, a precursor to anal cancer, the FDA extended its approval of Merck's vaccine, Gardasil, to include "the prevention of anal cancer and associated precancerous lesions . . . in people ages 9 through 26."[20] As stated in the FDA press release, "Although anal cancer is uncommon in the general population the incidence is increasing. HPV is associated with approximately 90 percent of anal cancer."[21] Thus, a connection between HPV and cancer among men was formally established, bringing forward boys as responsible to prevent genital warts and anal cancer. While anal cancer affects people of all genders, the cancer rates, and thus cancer burden, were higher for women compared to all men, yet MSM were emerging as a group at high risk for developing this cancer.[22] With this knowledge, renewed attempts to degender vaccination emerged as pharma and pediatrics shaped the "rightness" of the vaccine; the goal was no longer limited to "One Less" girl or woman with cervical cancer but expanded to include fewer boys and men with anal cancer, too. Given this cancer's association with anal sex, which often clings (despite the inaccuracy) to gay men's bodies and sexualities, it is of little surprise that, in contrast to vaccine introduction for girls and women, no DTC education or awareness campaigns preceded or followed these decisions to include boys. These omissions, we argue, are evidence of the complexity of degendering, the ways gender is always entangled with other social categories, and an early sign of a regendering (i.e., refeminizing) of HPV through reinforcement of an increased responsibility for cisgender girls and women.

In October 2011, however, ACIP issued a formal recommendation that the vaccine be routinely administered to boys ages eleven to twelve, with catchup vaccination up to age twenty-one in the general population or age twenty-six in MSM and people who are immunocompromised.[23] This made the United States the first country to implement a gender-neutral routine HPV vaccination strategy. Subsequent efforts to degender the vaccine began to emerge in DTC advertising depicting images of boys alongside girls, such as the 2011 Merck campaign, *Both*. The images in the *Both* campaign, similar to early campaigns, preempt a sex panic by discursively producing young teens as marked by their separation and sibling suggestion. An enclosed blue circle surrounds the headshots of presumably male bodies. "Your son [in blue type] or daughter [in red type] could be one [red] less [blue] person affected by HPV disease"; the circles for the headshots also formed the basis for the "male" and "female" symbols. The message was an inclusionary one, albeit a binary gendered one, where boys and girls share responsibility—with their parents—for the "right" job of vaccination, whether it be to achieve cancer prevention or something else. It is HPV disease that emerges as the object of health and, for boys, the source driving a moral responsibility to secure their own direct, yet unspecified, benefit.

Given the FDA's initial approval of the vaccine for only girls and women, based on data available at the time, and based on pharma selling it as a cervical cancer vaccine, boys and men remained absent from public discourse about the HPV vaccine. However, many public health experts had long hoped that all adolescents would be vaccinated in an effort to establish herd immunity.[24] Additionally, although historically cervical cancer had the highest number of new cases of all HPV-associated cancers, cervical cancer rates have been declining in the United States while rates of HPV-associated oropharyngeal and anal cancers have been increasing.[25] In fact, in the United States, there are now more new cases of HPV-associated oropharyngeal cancer per year (3,400 among women and 14,800 among men) than there are cervical cancer cases.[26]

Furthermore, the notion that vaccinating girls and women would be sufficient to protect boys and men hinges on the assumption that cisgender men engage in sex only with cisgender women, rendering MSM and trans people invisible. As sociologist Steven Epstein shows, during early debates over the gendering of HPV vaccination, a debate over access to the vaccine by gay men had simultaneously been suppressed due to the "undiscussable" nature of anal cancer.[27] Ultimately, the inclusion of boys and men in vaccination shed some light on this debate; it also resexualized the vaccine by revealing HPV's connection to anal cancer and focusing on MSM as an HPV risk group. For the most part, however, the connection between HPV and anal cancer remained absent from subsequent campaigns.

Efforts to incorporate boys into the HPV cancer prevention landscape have undoubtedly been made. Recent public health campaigns, which increasingly rely on social media and online video clips in lieu of TV commercials, exemplify this shift. For example, in 2018, Merck launched the *Versed* campaign, a possible attempt to correct for earlier gendering (and desexualizing) of HPV vaccines. The campaign incorporates young men in its imagery and, unlike early campaigns, describes HPV as a sexually transmitted virus. It acknowledges that "HPV doesn't discriminate. It can affect someone of any gender or sexual orientation."[28] This overt acknowledgment and shift from a cervical cancer vaccine to an STI vaccine, we and others argue, was necessary in order to degender the vaccine.[29] Yet *Versed* still does not, through its imagery or its text, explicitly address sexual activities, sidestepping attention to anal sex, even though anal sex is fairly common and is emerging as a practice that increases people's risk of anal cancer.[30]

In another move to include boys, in 2018, the American Cancer Society (ACS) announced the launch of its public health campaign, *Mission: HPV Cancer Free*, with a goal to reach 80 percent vaccination coverage for preteen boys and girls.[31] On the ACS homepage, a single photo of a child (presumably male) appears with the headline "HPV Vaccination Is Cancer Prevention" and an accompanying tagline, "Talk to your Healthcare Provider Today."[32] The volunteer organization is actively working to increase vaccination rates, especially among boys. When one clicks through these pages, the site speaks directly to parents—"Kids dream big . . . Give your kids a better chance of realizing those dreams"—and enrolls pediatricians. It encourages the viewing parent to "talk to your child's doctor" if the child is "near age 11." The images throughout depict young children, white-coated doctors, and, at times, parents. While these campaigns produce boys as holding some responsibility for HPV prevention, this responsibility is depicted as part of a collective effort including parents, peers, and doctors.

These efforts, it seems, have not been sufficient to degender HPV vaccination. While the gender gap in vaccination rates seems to be narrowing, rates among boys continue to lag in comparison to girls: in 2017, an estimated 62.6 percent of boys ages thirteen to seventeen had received one or more doses and 44.3 percent had received the recommended number of doses, compared to 68.6 percent and 53.1 percent, respectively, for girls the same age.[33]

Regendering HPV: Expanding Women's Responsibility

The same year that Merck launched the *Versed* campaign, the FDA approved use of the HPV vaccine through age forty-five in all genders. Yet this decision seemed to be chiefly based on data from women. As the 2018 FDA press release for expanded vaccination states, "Effectiveness of Gardasil 9 in men 27 through 45 years of age is inferred from the data described . . . in women 27 through 45 years of age, as well as efficacy data from Gardasil in younger men (16 through 26 years of age) and immunogenicity data from a clinical trial in which 150 men, 27 through 45 years of age, received a 3-dose regimen of Garda-sil."[34] Despite data inclusion and an announcement of age expansion of HPV vaccine eligibility for people of all genders, a subtle inequity persisted: although the vaccine was now approved for those through age forty-five, *routine vaccine recommendations* continued to be contingent on gender, with catchup vaccination recommended for women through age twenty-six but only through age twenty-one for most men (with the exception of MSM and immunocompromised persons, for whom the age twenty-six guideline applied). This means that women, MSM, and immunocompromised men continued to disproportionately carry the burden of vaccination, and it implies that certain groups are more impacted by HPV than others. A moral responsibility for health through vaccination is epidemiologically justified given current disease rates, yet misconstrues the message that *all* can be impacted by HPV and HPV-associated cancers. *All* are implicated actors in HPV transmission and thus *all* can have a role in disease prevention responsibility.

In June 2019, this gender inequity was eliminated when ACIP recommended "catch-up HPV vaccination for all persons through age 26 years," thereby including all men through age twenty-six as well.[35] While the call to harmonize age recommendations is justified by protection of a greater proportion of the population and the fact that men are also and, increasingly, impacted by HPV-associated cancers, some have suggested the decision was based on convenience. An *Associated Press* article noted that "the panel decided Wednesday to equalize the age recommendations to make it easier for doctors."[36] At the same meeting, and in line with the earlier FDA approval, ACIP recommended age expansion, although it recommended that people ages twenty-seven to forty-five should engage in shared decision making with their providers to determine if vaccination is right for them.[37] Notably, the updated recommendations do not offer guidance for clinicians to determine *who* among those aged twenty-seven to forty-five should (and should not) receive the vaccine, raising concerns among many ACIP members and mirroring, through implication, earlier recommendations that HPV vaccination was optional for boys.[38]

Given the recent date of these approvals, little is known about uptake of the HPV vaccine among adults ages twenty-seven to forty-five in the United States or about off-label use of the vaccine among men and especially MSM in the early years.[39] However, research confirms that the vaccine is most effective when administered prior to sexual debut (or HPV exposure) and that the greatest vaccination impact has been on disease prevalence among younger age groups.[40] Therefore, the future enrollment in and impact of vaccination for older age groups is unknown. In theory, these policy changes harmonize gender differences in vaccine recommendations, thereby completing the degendering process. But, in practice, it is not clear that they equalize the burden of vaccination and burden of HPV-associated cancers. We argue that they do not, in fact, eliminate the gender inequity in the responsibility to get vaccinated and that a regendering of HPV (i.e., realignment with femininity) has emerged. As a result, women continue to hold the burden for HPV-associated cancer prevention as primary vaccine and secondary screening prevention tools conjoin as the "right tools" for cervical cancer prevention.

Despite efforts to incorporate boys into DTC advertising and public health campaign goals, these efforts have so far been insufficient to degender HPV vaccination, as evidenced by the continued gender gap in vaccination. Associations between gender and vaccination have not mobilized the same moral responsibility for boys and men to receive the vaccine. Parents of boys have lower odds of reporting that their child's provider/pediatrician recommended the HPV vaccine, which, in turn, is cited as a reason for lack of vaccination, particularly among boys.[41] This inherently places a greater responsibility burden on girls than it does on boys. Whereas girls are expected to receive the vaccine, that expectation remains weaker for boys; nor, until recently, was the age range for vaccination as expansive for men as for women. Although men's incorporation into routine vaccine recommendations implies some degree of self-responsibility for one's health, depictions of agency and choice for boys and men have been dim in both U.S. policy recommendations and Merck advertisements. For example, only one state school vaccination mandate, in Rhode Island, includes boys and girls.[42] In more recent DTC promotional materials, boys and men are now central actors, yet unlike the girls of *One Less*, the boys in the *Versed* campaign do not hold signs or make declarations, instead passively presenting information: "Did you know that 75 percent of men can get HPV in their lifetime?" "Did you know that Gardasil was approved by the Food and Drug Administration (FDA) for use in boys and young men ages 9 to 26 to help protect against 90 percent of genital warts cases?" The connection between infection and disease is less clear, and the action plan is absent.

Perhaps this lack of clarity is due to the murkiness surrounding HPV vaccine as the "right tool" for the job among boys. What, after all, is the "job"? As we have demonstrated, over the course of efforts to incorporate boys in vaccination, various arguments for doing so have been put forth—direct risk of genital warts, direct risk of anal cancer, and promotion of herd immunity. These various targets of prevention beg the question of what "job" the vaccine is intended to fill for boys and men: Is the job to help protect girls and women from cervical cancer? Or is it to protect boys and men in their own right? This isn't to say a multiplicity of objects of prevention are not possible but rather to suggest that the job remains murky to the public, resulting in many guardians questioning why their sons should be vaccinated and a target of continued public engagement with vaccination efforts.

In contrast, women historically have carried more of the burden for HPV-related cancer prevention, as cervical cancer remains the most visible object of HPV cancer prevention despite rising rates of other HPV-related cancers. Thus far, we have argued that this is due to the gendered claims-making of HPV policy guidelines, marketing, and popular media coverage of the HPV vaccine. However, it is also in part attributable to HPV-associated cancer screening technologies that are currently available and, as we will speculate, seems unlikely to change despite recent vaccination guideline changes. While the HPV vaccine is merely one approach in a toolkit used to prevent cervical cancer among women, the same is not true for men, for whom no routine HPV-related screening approach is nationally recommended. Although anal cancer screening is available, it is not routinely recommended, although some clinical experts recommend screening in high-risk populations, such as people living with HIV or previous anogenital cancers or, at times, MSM. Cervical cancer screening, in the form of either Pap testing and/or HPV testing, is the only HPV-associated cancer screening supported by professional organization guidelines. This demonstrates how pediatrics continues to shape health care in uneven and gendered ways. Women have a moral responsibility *both* to receive the HPV vaccine, ideally in adolescence, for the herd *and* to seek cervical cancer screening for later-in-life direct benefit in accordance with professional guidelines.

While we anticipate integration of these approaches, professional organizations have yet to couple HPV vaccination and cervical cancer screening guidelines into a single approach.[43] It remains unknown if or how vaccination (or vaccination status) will be integrated into the existing cervical cancer screening paradigm. However, given that HPV vaccination protects against only certain types of HPV, leaving recipients susceptible to cervical cancer (although to a far lesser degree), we expect screening to continue, although perhaps with modified and stratified recommendations. Already, this message increasingly appears in ads and public health campaigns. For example, on the *Versed* website, the final question on a mini quiz is, "I always use condoms, All good then?"[44] The response states, "Condoms only cover so much. HPV can affect areas that aren't covered. . . . There are other ways to protect yourself, like abstinence, limiting the number of sexual partners you have, and, for women, routine cervical cancer screenings." This approach is one piece of a larger societal phenomenon in which cisgender women are expected to regularly seek preventive health care and engage in conversations about sex with their provider, whereas this expectation does not (yet) exist for heterosexual men. However, we do see parallels among MSM, who are also expected to more routinely engage in care, particularly STI testing, than are heterosexual men, as well as people living with HIV, who are expected to maintain engagement in care and who have been identified as high-risk populations for HPV-associated disease. This is relevant not only as we consider screening but also in light of the recent vaccine age expansion: if (heterosexual) men are not routinely seeking care, when will they be offered the HPV vaccine?

Cisgender women are further burdened as organizations and media articles continue to emphasize not only the connection between HPV and cervical cancer but also the possibility of eliminating cervical cancer. In May 2018, the director-general of the World Health Organization made a call for the global elimination of cervical cancer, referring to it as "one of the greatest threats to women's health." "Our challenge is to ensure that all girls globally are vaccinated against HPV and that every woman over 30 is screened and treated for pre-cancerous lesions," he said.[45]

Conclusion: The Politics of HPV Claims-Making

The HPV vaccine's story calls to mind not so much the vaccine markets of the early twentieth century, which targeted children susceptible to highly contagious and life-threatening diseases, but a twenty-first-century pharmaceutical industry approach that markets directly to consumers by appealing to personal ideals of individual choice and expression, responsibility and empowerment, and self-care and enhancement.[46] Its administration to preadolescents reveals the ways pediatrics has "always been involved in social, political, and cultural questions beyond the domain of the sickbed, clinic, and hospital."[47] In the evolving case of HPV vaccination, pediatrics gets entangled in public health and adult health care through vaccination policy, promotion, and marketing. Vaccination rates have variously hinged on the ways gender (as well as sexuality) are managed. The HPV vaccine first aligned with femininity inscribed into technologies associated with sexual and reproductive health. Processes to degender HPV and HPV vaccination proved challenging and seem to have been met with a regendering of HPV: women are reminded that they are responsible for the herd *and* for reducing their individual risk of cervical cancer through screening programs.

Further, the burden of HPV-associated cancer prevention is not equally imposed on all people with cervices. Emphasis on "womanhood" and "protecting women" continues to render trans and nonconforming people—children or adult—invisible in the realm of cervical cancer prevention, exacerbating inequities already experienced by these populations. Additionally, there is often a misperception that women engaging in sex with women are at lower risk of HPV and therefore have less of a need to seek cervical cancer screening. Dispelling this inaccuracy is gradually taking place with headlines such as "Don't believe the myth: lesbians can get HPV."[48] Interventions have also increasingly targeted subgroups of women historically disproportionately burdened by cervical cancer and/or with lower screening rates, including Black and Latina women, immigrants, and women living in rural regions of the United States, with increasing attention paid to the intersections of these social categories.[49]

Yet while these efforts seem to focus on women, the HPV vaccine is a(n) (ideally) childhood vaccine intended to protect adolescents from an STI that *might* result in disease during adulthood. The continued coupling of the HPV vaccine with cervical cancer and women's health obfuscates the fact that the vaccine is principally intended to reduce *risk* of disease—cancer caused by HPV infection—rather than prevent disease itself. Although "cancer prevention was neither an established component of pediatric care nor an accepted health responsibility of the nation's youngest citizens,"[50] introduction of the HPV vaccine and, particularly, selling it as a cancer prevention vaccine resulted in added responsibility for pediatricians and adolescents, particularly adolescent girls. We have yet to see the societal impact of harmonizing the HPV vaccine age recommendation across genders. However, as we have demonstrated, while an action plan for girls and women remains clear (vaccination plus screening) and the setting in which this should occur has been defined (pediatric and gynecologic offices), an action plan for men, especially heterosexual men, seems to be absent, implying their lesser moral responsibility. We are not arguing for a degendered, desexualized approach to HPV vaccination that sanitizes sexuality and erases differences along categories of age, race/ethnicity, place of childhood, and health care experience, among other social categories. But we are advocating for equity over equality: a health care approach that acknowledges differences in vulnerabilities, exposures, and health care needs while also advocating for structural changes that ensure more equitable distribution of needed health protection. The new vaccination plus screening strategy is in and of itself a highly stratified approach, and it remains to be revealed who the epistemic and ontological objects will be and who stands to benefit. We reject high investments in populations and places least burdened by disease and instead advocate for an approach that accounts for differences in health and illness.

Notes

1. While "sex" and "gender" are socially produced, malleable terms, we deploy these terms in the language of pharma, policy, and pediatrics when referring to the documents analyzed for this chapter. We understand gender as a social process and a social category in our analysis.

2. Nelly Oudshoorn, *The Male Pill: A Biography of a Technology in the Making* (Durham, NC: Duke University Press, 2003).

3. Adele E. Clarke et al., eds., *Biomedicalization: Technoscience, Health, and Illness in the U.S.* (Durham, NC: Duke University Press, 2010), 63; Robert Crawford, "Healthism and the Medicalization of Everyday Life," *International Journal of Health Service* 10, no. 3 (1980): 365–88; Deborah Lupton, *The Imperative of Health: Public Health and the Regulated Body* (Thousand Oaks, CA: Sage, 1995); Jonathan Metzl and Anna Kirkland, eds., *Against Health: How Health Became the New Morality* (New York: NYU Press, 2010); Nikolas Rose, *The Politics of Life Itself: Biomedicine, Power, and Subjectivity in the Twenty-First Century* (Princeton, NJ: Princeton University Press, 2007).

4. We focus on the Gardasil vaccine, manufactured by Merck & Co., because this HPV vaccine formulation has come to dominate the U.S. market.

5. Age-standardized cervical cancer rates and the proportion of cancers attributable to cervical cancer vary greatly worldwide. See Catherine de Martel et al., "Worldwide Burden of Cancer Attributable to HPV by Site, Country and HPV Type," *International Journal of Cancer* 141, no. 4 (August 2017): 664–70; Freddie Bray et al., "Global Cancer Statistics 2018: GLOBOCAN Estimates of Incidence and Mortality Worldwide for 36 Cancers in 185 Countries," *CA: A Cancer Journal for Clinicians* 68, no. 6 (November 2018): 394–424. However, in the United States, cervical cancer is fairly uncommon; see ACS, *Cancer Facts & Figures 2019* (Atlanta: American Cancer Society, 2019).

6. Clarke and Fujimura argue that "tools," "jobs," and "rightness" are co-constructed in developing social problems and strategies to address those problems. Rightness is not a property of a tool but rather results from interactions; see Adele E. Clarke and Joan H. Fujimura, "What Tools? Which Jobs? Why Right?" in *The Right Tools for the Job: At Work in Twentieth-Century Life Sciences*, ed. Adele E. Clarke and Joan H. Fujimura (Princeton, NJ: Princeton University Press, 1992), 3–44.

7. Sarah H. Landis et al., "Cancer Statistics, 1999," *CA: A Cancer Journal for Clinicians* 49, no. 1 (1999): 8–31.

8. Stuart Blume, *Immunization: How Vaccines Became Controversial* (London: Reaktion Books, 2017).

9. Monica J. Casper and Laura M. Carpenter, "Sex, Drugs, and Politics: The HPV Vaccine for Cervical Cancer," *Sociology of Health & Illness* 30, no. 6 (September 2008): 886–99; Ellen M. Daley et al., "The Feminization of HPV: How Science, Politics, Economics and Gender Norms Shaped U.S. HPV Vaccine Implementation," *Papillomavirus Research* 3 (2017): 142–48; Samantha D. Gottlieb, *Not Quite a Cancer Vaccine: Selling HPV and Cervical Cancer* (New Brunswick, NJ: Rutgers University Press, 2018); Keith Wailoo et al., eds., *Three Shots at Prevention: The HPV Vaccine and the Politics of Medicine's Simple Solutions* (Baltimore, MD: Johns Hopkins University Press, 2010).

10. Elena Conis, "'Do We Really Need Hepatitis B on the Second Day of Life?' Vaccination Mandates and Shifting Representations of Hepatitis B," *Journal of Medical Humanities* 32, no. 2 (June 2011): 155–66; Mamo and Epstein, "The Pharmaceuticalization of Sexual Risk," *Social Science & Medicine* 101 (January 2014): 155–65.

11. Wailoo et al., *Three Shots at Prevention.*

12. Laura Mamo, Amber Nelson, and Aleia Clark, "Producing and Protecting Risky Girlhoods," in *Three Shots at Prevention: The HPV Vaccine and the Politics of Medicine's Simple Solutions*, ed. Keith Wailoo et al. (Baltimore, MD: Johns Hopkins University Press, 2010), 121–45; Elena Conis, *Vaccine Nation: America's Changing Relationship with Immunization* (Chicago: University of Chicago Press, 2015), 227–49.

13. Adele E. Clarke and Monica J. Casper, "From Simple Technology to Complex Arena: Classification of Pap Smears, 1917–90," *Medical Anthropology Quarterly* 10, no. 4 (December 1996): 601–23.

14. Christina G. Dorell et al., "Human Papillomavirus Vaccination Series Initiation and Completion, 2008–2009," *Pediatrics* 128, no. 5 (November 2011): 830–39.

15. Vicki B. Benard et al., "Timeliness of Cervical Cancer Diagnosis and Initiation of Treatment in the National Breast and Cervical Cancer Early Detection Program," *Journal of Women's Health* 21, no. 7 (July 2012): 776–82; Centers for Disease Control and Prevention (CDC), "HPV-Associated Cervical Cancer Rates by Race/Ethnicity," last reviewed August 20, 2018, https://www.cdc.gov/cancer/hpv/statistics/cervical.htm.

16. Mamo and Epstein, "The Pharmaceuticalization of Sexual Risk," 155–65.

17. Tanja Y. Walker et al., "National, Regional, State, and Selected Local Area Vaccination Coverage among Adolescents Aged 13–17 Years—United States, 2017," *Morbidity and Mortality Weekly Report* 67, no. 33 (August 24, 2018): 909–17.

18. CDC, "FDA Licensure of Quadrivalent Human Papillomavirus Vaccine (HPV4, Gardasil) for Use in Males and Guidance from the Advisory Committee on Immunization Practices (ACIP)," *Morbidity and Mortality Weekly Report* 59, no. 20 (May 28, 2010): 630–32.

19. CDC, "FDA Licensure of Quadrivalent Human Papillomavirus Vaccine (HPV4, Gardasil) for Use in Males," 630–32. ACIP is a committee comprising medical and public health experts who develop vaccine use recommendations for the effective control of vaccine-preventable diseases in the United States.

20. FDA, "FDA News Release: Gardasil Approved to Prevent Anal Cancer," December 22, 2010, https://www.prnewswire.com/news-releases/fda-gardasil-approved-to-prevent-anal-cancer-112326644.html.

21. FDA, "Gardasil Approved to Prevent Anal Cancer."

22. There are about 4,300 new cases of HPV-associated anal cancer among women and 2,200 new cases among men diagnosed each year in the United States; see CDC, "HPV-Associated Anal Cancer Rates by Race and Ethnicity," last reviewed August 20, 2018, https://www.cdc.gov/cancer/hpv/statistics/anal.htm. In addition to MSM, people living with HIV and other immunocompromised conditions and people with previous reproductive cancers are emerging as population groups at higher risk of developing anal cancer compared to the general population. Andrew E. Grulich et al., "Incidence of Cancers in People with HIV/AIDS Compared with Immunosuppressed Transplant Recipients: A Meta-Analysis," *The Lancet* 370, no. 9581 (July 2007): 59–67; ACS, "Risk Factors for Anal Cancer," https://www.cancer.org/cancer/anal-cancer/causes-risks-prevention/risk-factors.html (accessed July 29, 2019).

23. CDC, "Recommendations on the Use of Quadrivalent Human Papillomavirus Vaccine in Males—Advisory Committee on Immunization Practices (ACIP), 2011," *Morbidity and Mortality Weekly Report* 60, no. 50 (December 23, 2011): 1705–8; Jane J. Kim, "Targeted Human Papillomavirus Vaccination of Men Who Have Sex with Men in the USA: A Cost-Effectiveness Modelling Analysis," *The Lancet Infectious*

Diseases 10, no. 12 (December 2010): 845–52. MSM and immunocompromised peo-ple had a higher age of vaccine eligibility because evidence showed that this was cost-effective given their higher risk of anal cancer and genital warts compared to the general population.

24. For example, see Karin B. Michels and Harald zur Hausen, "HPV Vaccine for All," *The Lancet* 374, no. 9686 (July 2009): 268–70.

25. There are "six [HPV-associated] cancers" often invoked in HPV prevention messages: cervical, vulvar, vaginal, anal, throat (oropharyngeal), and penial cancers; see Amer-ican Cancer Society (ACS), "American Cancer Society Launches Campaign to Elimi-nate Cervical Cancer. Mission: HPV Cancer Free Aims to Increase Vaccination Rates Among Boys and Girls to 80 percent," June 6, 2018, http://pressroom.cancer.org/HPV-cancerfreelaunch. For information about trends, see Elizabeth A. Van Dyne, S. Jane Henley, Mona Saraiya, Cheryll C. Thomas, Lauri E. Markowitz, and Vicki B. Benard, "Trends in Human Papillomavirus–Associated Cancers—United States, 1999–2015," *Morbidity and Mortality Weekly Report* 67, no. 33 (August 24, 2018): 918–24.

26. ACS, *Cancer Facts & Figures 2019*.

27. Steven Epstein, "The Great Undiscussable: HPV, Anal Cancer, and Gay Men's Health," in *Three Shots at Prevention: The HPV Vaccine and the Politics of Medicine's Simple Solutions*, ed. Keith Wailoo, Julie Livingston, Steven Epstein, and Robert Aronow-itz (Baltimore, MD: Johns Hopkins University Press, 2010), 61–90.

28. *Versed*, Merck Sharp & Dohme Corp., last revised July 2018, https://www.versedhpv .com/.

29. Conis, *Vaccine Nation*, 227–49.

30. Debby Herbenick et al., "Sexual Behavior in the United States: Results from a National Probability Sample of Men and Women Ages 14–94," *Journal of Sexual Medicine* 7 (October 2010): 255–65; SKYN Condoms by Lifestyles, "2017 SKYN® Condoms Millennial Sex Survey Reveals Nearly 50 percent of Respondents Sext at Least Once a Week," *PR Newswire*, February 6, 2017, https://www.prnewswire.com/news -releases/2017-skyn-condoms-millennial-sex-survey-reveals-nearly-50-of-respon dents-sext-at-least-once-a-week-300401985.html; ACS, "Risk Factors for Anal Cancer."

31. ACS, "American Cancer Society Launches Campaign to Eliminate Cervical Cancer."

32. ACS, https://www.cancer.org/ (accessed July 29, 2019). Note that the ACS homep-age seems to rotate images. This was merely one version of the page on the date the website was accessed.

33. Walker et al., "National, Regional, State, and Selected Local Area Vaccination Cov-erage," 909–17.

34. FDA, "FDA Approved Expanded Use of Gardasil 9 to Include Individuals 27 through 45 Years Old," October 5, 2018, https://www.fda.gov/news-events/press-announce ments/fda-approves-expanded-use-gardasil-9-include-individuals-27-through -45-years-old.

35. Elissa Meites et al., "Human Papillomavirus Vaccination for Adults: Updated Rec-ommendations of the Advisory Committee on Immunization Practices," *Morbidity and Mortality Weekly Report* 68, no. 32 (August 16, 2019), 698.

36. Mike Strobe, "Vaccine Panel Gives Nod to HPV Shots for Men Up to Age 26," *The Associated Press*, June 26, 2019, https://www.apnews.com/e341072cbfa040369fd 157bd255ed40a.

37. Meites et al., "Human Papillomavirus Vaccination for Adults," 700.

38. Ashley Lyles, "ACIP: HPV, Pneumococcal Vax Guidelines Revised—Panel Empha-sizes Shared Decision-Making," *MedPage Today*, June 27, 2019, https://www.med pagetoday.com/meetingcoverage/acip/80728.

39. Off-label use (administration of the vaccine that is not in accordance with vaccina-tion guidelines) has been anecdotally reported in the United States, particularly among MSM. This first occurred when the HPV vaccine was given to men before the vaccine was formally approved for use in boys and men. Later, there were reports that MSM regardless of age were vaccinated in some clinics. For example, see Kris-tin A. Swedish and Stephen E. Goldstone, "Prevention of Anal Condyloma with Quadrivalent Human Papillomavirus Vaccination of Older Men Who Have Sex with Men," *PLoS One* 9, no. 4 (April 2014): e93393.

40. Mélanie Drolet et al., "Population-Level Impact and Herd Effects following the Intro-duction of Human Papillomavirus Vaccination Programmes: Updated Systematic Review and Meta-Analysis," *The Lancet* 394, no. 10197 (August 2019): 497–509.

41. Kahee A. Mohammed et al., "Disparities in Provider Recommendation of Human Pap-illomavirus Vaccination for US Adolescents," *Journal of Adolescent Health* 59, no. 5 (November 2016): 592–98; Megan C. Lindley et al., "Comparing Human Papillomavi-rus Vaccine Knowledge and Intentions among Parents of Boys and Girls," *Human Vaccines & Immunotherapeutics* 12, no. 6 (2016): 1519–27.

42. Only three U.S. jurisdictions—Rhode Island, Virginia, and Washington, D.C.—have school mandates at present. Our point persists nonetheless.

43. This is not to say that cervical cancer screening guidelines have not changed since HPV vaccine introduction. Since the vaccine was introduced, screening guidelines have changed to recommend cotesting (i.e., use of both cervical cytology and HPV test-ing) in lieu of cervical cytology alone among those aged thirty to sixty-five years. More recently, the U.S. Preventive Services Task Force approved HPV testing alone (every three years) as an acceptable form of screening among those aged thirty to sixty-five years; see Susan J. Curry et al., "Screening for Cervical Cancer: US Preventive Services Task Force Recommendation Statement," *JAMA* 320, no. 7 (August 2018): 674–86. However, HPV vaccination has not been integrated into these guidelines, although Bosch et al. offer one example of how this might be accomplished; see F. Xavier Bosch et al., "HPV-FASTER: Broadening the Scope for Prevention of HPV-Related Cancer," *Nature Reviews Clinical Oncology* 13, no. 2 (February 2016): 119–32.

44. *Versed*, Merck Sharp & Dohme Corp.

45. Tedros Adhanom Ghebreyesus, "Cervical Cancer: An NCD We Can Overcome," WHO, Intercontinental Hotel, Geneva, May 19, 2018, https://www.who.int/reproductivehe alth/DG_Call-to-Action.pdf.

46. Mamo et al., "Producing and Protecting Risky Girlhoods," 121–45; Robert A. Aronow-itz, "Vaccines against Cancer," in *Three Shots at Prevention: The HPV Vaccine and the Politics of Medicine's Simple Solutions*, ed. Keith Wailoo et al. (Baltimore, MD: Johns Hopkins University Press, 2010), 21–38.

47. Alexandra Minna Stern and Howard Markel, eds., *Formative Years: Children's Health in the United States 1880–2000* (Ann Arbor: University of Michigan Press, 2002), 1.

48. Gwendolyn Smith, "Don't Believe the Myth: Lesbians Can Get HPV," *LGBTQ Nation*, July 1, 2019, https://www.lgbtqnation.com/2019/07/dont-believe-myth-lesbians-can -get-hpv/.

49. Mita Sanghavi Goel et al., "Racial and Ethnic Disparities in Cancer Screening: The Importance of Foreign Birth as a Barrier to Care," *Journal of General Internal*

Medicine 18, no. 12 (December 2003): 1028–35; Gopal K. Singh et al., "Socioeconomic, Rural-Urban, and Racial Inequalities in US Cancer Mortality: Part I—All Cancers and Lung Cancer and Part II—Colorectal, Prostate, Breast, and Cervical Cancers," *Journal of Cancer Epidemiology* 12 (2011): 1–27.

50. Conis, *Vaccine Nation*, 232.

Notes on Contributors

Kathleen E. Bachynski is an assistant professor of public health at Muhlenberg College. She researches and teaches on topics in sports safety, epidemiology, public health ethics, and history of medicine. She is the author of *No Game for Boys to Play: The History of Youth Football and the Origins of a Public Health Crisis* (2019).

Elena Conis, a historian specializing in the history of public health, medicine, and the public understanding of science, is an associate professor in the Graduate School of Journalism and Center for Science, Technology, Medicine, and Society at the University of California, Berkeley. She is the author of *Vaccine Nation: America's Changing Relationship with Immunization* (2015).

Sandra Eder is an assistant professor in the history department at the University of California, Berkeley, where she teaches U.S. gender history and the history of medicine. Her research focuses on gender and sexuality in medicine and science, clinical practices and patient records, and the science of happiness. She is currently completing a book manuscript on the emergence of the sex/gender binary in mid-twentieth-century American medicine. She has published in *Gender & History*, *Endeavour*, and the *Bulletin of the History of Medicine*.

Hughes Evans is Marcus Professor of General Pediatrics and Adolescent Medicine at Emory University. She directs the division of general pediatrics and adolescent medicine and is active in medical student and resident education. Her current research is on attitudes about Down syndrome in mid-twentieth-century America.

Jules Gill-Peterson is an assistant professor of English and gender, sexuality, and women's studies at the University of Pittsburgh, where she researches transgender studies, trans of color theory, and the history of science and medicine. She is the author of *Histories of the Transgender Child* (2018), winner of a Lambda Literary Award for Transgender Nonfiction.

Jessica Martucci earned her PhD in the history and sociology of science in 2011 from the University of Pennsylvania. She has published numerous academic and popular works on motherhood, science, and disability, including her book *Back to the Breast: Natural Motherhood and Breastfeeding in America* (2015). She is a research associate in the Department of Medical Humanities and Ethics at Columbia University.

Laura Mamo is Health Equity Institute Professor of Health Education at San Francisco State University. She is a sociologist of science, technology, and medicine whose research examines cultural, social, and political entanglements of gender and sexuality with science, medicine, and health. She is the author of *Queering Reproduction: Achieving Pregnancy in the Age of Technoscience* (2007); coeditor of *Biomedicalization: Technoscience, Health, and Illness in the U.S.* (2010); and coauthor of *Living Green: Communities That Sustain* (2009). Her current research examines the crossroads of sexually transmitted viruses and cancers, with a focus on the gendered and sexual politics and biomedicalization of HPV.

Aimee Medeiros is an associate professor in the Department of Humanities and Social Sciences at the University of California, San Francisco. She is the author of *Heightened Expectations: The Rise of the Human Growth Hormone Industry in America* (2016). She specializes in the history of pediatrics, gender studies, and science and technology studies.

Christine H. Morton is a medical sociologist in the Division of Neonatal and Developmental Medicine in the pediatrics department at Stanford University. She researches maternal mortality and morbidity and collaborates with clinical and public health stakeholders in translating findings into quality toolkits. Her work explores social meanings of maternal health quality among all stakeholders. She is the author of *Birth Ambassadors: Doulas and the Re-emergence of Woman-Supported Childbirth in America* (2014) and founded ReproNetwork.org, an international listserv with over 600 subscribers, mostly social scientists interested in reproductive/maternal practices, policies, and ideologies.

Ashley E. Pérez is a doctoral candidate in sociology at the University of California, San Francisco and a research associate at the Health Equity Institute at San Francisco State University. Her research focuses on gender, sexual orientation, and racial/ethnic inequities in sexual health and cancer prevention. She received her bachelor's and master's degrees from Brown University and has published in journals such as the *American Journal of Preventive Medicine, Journal of Women's Health*, and *LGBT Health*.

Heather Munro Prescott is a professor of history and Connecticut State University Professor at Central Connecticut State University. Her research interests include U.S. women's history, history of childhood, and disability history. She is the author of *The Morning After: A History of Emergency Contraception in the United States* (Rutgers University Press, 2011), *Student Bodies: The Impact of Student Health on American Society and Medicine* (2007), and *A Doctor of Their Own: The History of Adolescent Medicine* (1998).

Jochen Profit graduated from the University of Freiburg Medical School and completed his Neonatology and Health Services Research training at Harvard. Since 2013, he has been on the faculty at Stanford, where he is currently associate professor of pediatrics and chief quality officer of the California Perinatal Quality Care Collaborative. His research, funded by the National Institutes of Health and other federal, foundation, and intramural sources, focuses on the optimization of quality of neonatal-perinatal health care delivery. He has served various national scientific and professional organization panels, including the National Academy of Sciences and the National Institutes of Health.

A. R. Ruis is a historian of medicine and public health and a learning scientist at the University of Wisconsin–Madison. He studies the history of food and nutrition and the use of quantitative techniques to model rich qualitative data. He is the author of *Eating to Learn, Learning to Eat: The Origins of School Lunch in the United States* (Rutgers University Press, 2017).

Krista Sigurdson is a postdoctoral research fellow in the Division of Neonatal and Developmental Medicine in the pediatrics department at Stanford University. She is a medical sociologist and science and technology studies scholar whose work focuses on the intersection of child and maternal health. Her previous work focused on the sociology of infant feeding, specifically the exchange of human milk via milk banking, milk sharing, and scientific enterprise. Her current work concerns the quality of hospital neonatal care particularly vis-à-vis racial and ethnic disparities in care and/or family experiences of care.

Index

Available titles in the Critical Issues in Health and Medicine series: